LOW BLOOD SUGAR

By the same author:

DIETS TO HELP DIABETES
DIETS TO HELP MIGRAINE
RECIPES FOR HEALTH: LOW BLOOD SUGAR
(with Maggie Budd)

LOW BLOOD SUGAR

COPING WITH LOW BLOOD SUGAR
(HYPOGLYCAEMIA)

Martin Budd
D.O., M.R.O., Lic.Ac.

Thorsons
An Imprint of HarperCollinsPublishers

While the creators of this work have made every effort to ensure that the information presented is as accurate and up-to-date as possible at the time of publication, medical and pharmaceutical knowledge is constantly changing and the application of it to particular circumstances depends on many factors. Therefore readers are urged always to consult a qualified medical specialist for individual advice. This book should not be used as an alternative to appropriate medical care. The author and publishers cannot be held liable for any errors and omissions, or actions that may be taken as a result of using it.

Thorsons
An Imprint of HarperCollins*Publishers*
77–85 Fulham Palace Road,
Hammersmith, London W6 8JB

Published by Thorsons 1981
Second edition, revised and enlarged, 1984
Third edition, revised and updated, 1995
Reprinted 1997
3 5 7 9 10 8 6 4

A catalogue record for this book
is available from the British Library

ISBN 0 7225 3119 2

Printed and bound in Great Britain by
Caledonian International Book Manufacturing Ltd, Glasgow

CONTENTS

Note to reader

Before following the self-help advice given in this book readers are earnestly urged to give careful consideration to the nature of their particular health problem, and to consult a competent physician if in any doubt. This book should not be regarded as a substitute for professional medical treatment, and whilst every care is taken to ensure the accuracy of the content, the author and the publishers cannot accept legal responsibility for any problem arising out of the experimentation with the methods described.

Acknowledgement

My special thanks must go to Keith Lamont who introduced me to the diagnosis and treatment of low blood sugar over 20 years ago. His particular interest in glucose tolerance testing and enzyme testing has inspired many of his colleagues to a more empirical approach to nutritional medicine.

INTRODUCTION

Why is low blood sugar a common problem when many people eat far too much sugar? Why do sufferers from high blood sugar (diabetes or hyperglycaemia) and low blood sugar (hypoglycaemia) have to follow similar diets when their problems seem to be opposite? (N.B. The terms 'hypo' and 'hyper' which recur throughout the text mean 'too little' and 'too much' respectively.) Is sugar good for us or harmful, and does it really matter whether the sugar we eat is brown or white? How can sugar affect our memory and concentration and even our personalities? Are honey and molasses also sugars or harmless natural substitutes? What is the connection between low blood sugar and such diverse complaints as alcoholism, migraine, asthma, depression, arthritis, obesity and epilepsy? What is the relationship between sugar and fat, and does sugar really provide all our energy needs? What is the difference between reactive hypoglycaemia, functional hypoglycaemia and relative hypoglycaemia?

When discussing hypoglycaemia with patients, or when lecturing, I have frequently been asked similar questions, perhaps because hypoglycaemia is a confusing, complex and contradictory disease. In this book, I set out to answer these and other questions.

Although officially 'discovered' in 1924 by Seale Harris, an American physician, the medical establishment insists that hypoglycaemia is an extremely rare condition and that the functional hypoglycaemia due to faulty diet is a trendy condition invented by health-food faddists. Some nutritionists and scientists claim that hypoglycaemia is a temporary, easily-rectified imbalance; others see it as the basis of many serious diseases, a contributing factor to cancer, heart disease, diabetes, asthma and arthritis, etc.

Definitions of hypoglycaemia range from 'the opposite of diabetes' (hyperinsulinism) to the less simplistic view that blood sugar deficiency is due to complex interactions between the glandular, nervous and digestive systems. Even the diagnosis of hypoglycaemia is a subject of controversy. Many practitioners feel that a six-hour glucose tolerance test is a satisfactory and conclusive method of diagnosing hypoglycaemia. Others consider the test to be misleading and ambiguous and prefer to base their diagnosis on careful assessments of the patient's history and symptoms.

Perhaps you can begin to understand why I consider hypoglycaemia to be confusing and contradictory. It is perhaps unfortunate that the major symptoms of hypoglycaemia, e.g. fatigue, depression, headache and neurotic behaviour, are often diagnosed as being due to stress. Even in the second half of the twentieth century most doctors insist on the separation of disorders of the mind and body. It may well be that hypoglycaemia is the bridge which links many mental and physical symptoms, and that correct nutrition is the key to both.

1

SYMPTOMS OF HYPOGLYCAEMIA

Hypoglycaemia means literally low (hypo) blood sugar (glycaemia), or an abnormally low level of glucose in the blood. This definition is deceptively simple for it is possible to have symptoms of low blood sugar with a *normal* fasting level of sugar in the blood. Quite obviously the actual level of blood sugar is, by itself, an insufficient basis for the diagnosis of hypoglycaemia. This paradox will be explained later in the book in Chapter 11, on diagnosis. Another problem with the diagnosis of hypoglycaemia is that almost all the symptoms of hypoglycaemia can be caused by other pathological conditions.

General Indications

To discuss the diversity of symptoms causes by low blood sugar would take up most of the book. The list below, however is a representative selection of the most common symptoms:

Fatigue	Anxiety	Depression
Irritability	Forgetfulness	Poor concentration

Indigestion	Breathlessness	Panic feelings
Headaches	Migraine	Asthma
Overweight	Food cravings	Excessive smoking
Alcoholism	Vertigo	Sweating
Pre-menstrual tension	Muscular stiffness	Phobias
Numbness	Blurred vision	Cold extremities
Joint pain	Fainting and blackouts	Convulsions
Nightmares	Lack of sex drive	Allergies
Heart disease	Angina	Suicidal tendencies
Epilepsy	Stomach cramps	Stomach ulcers
Hyperactivity	Neuralgia	Agoraphobia
	Narcolepsy	Tinnitus

I am sure there will be many eyebrows raised at the great variety and number of symptoms mentioned and, at first sight, it is difficult to imagine that there is a common theme to all these conditions. (All this could be a hypochondriac's dream come true! He can tell his friends with a certain pride that he has hypoglycaemia and wait for the murmurings of sympathy.) Interestingly enough, many of the symptoms of low blood sugar are classed by doctors as 'stress disorders' and I hope to show, by describing the effect of sugar on the nervous system, that many of these symptoms are in fact due to nutritional imbalances and not personality failings. You may also see several of your own symptoms on the list; but simply to scan this list, recognize one's own symptoms and diagnose low blood sugar is clearly not the answer. As previously stated, many of these symptoms may have other causes, not least of which *could* be stress. It is therefore essential, in order to accurately diagnose hypoglycaemia, that more objective diagnostic methods be used. These include detailed case history taking and the six-hour glucose tolerance test.

At some time in their lives most people experience one or more of these symptoms. This is usually due to transient hypoglycaemia, which is defined as a temporary or passing drop in blood sugar level, and this is soon rectified by the body's own sugar regulation mechanism. Once a balance is achieved, the symptoms usually disappear. If, however, there is a real long-term imbalance in the sugar regulation the symptoms may well disappear or change, but they will always return unless the actual imbalance is corrected.

Now let us look more closely at the way in which a drop in the blood sugar directly affects the various organs and systems of the body, giving rise to the symptoms listed above. In this way you will begin to understand why the blood sugar level is so important to the normal running of the body. The effects can be classified as follows:

Nervous System Changes

The main nutrient needed by the nervous system is glucose. There is no really adequate substitute and, although other substances are involved, they cannot replace glucose. Unfortunately, it is not fully understood just how glucose acts on the nervous system, but it has been noted that when a healthy patient is injected with insulin (the opposite of glucose), there occurs, within minutes, profound and sudden changes in the efficiency of the nervous system. This is completely reversed by an injection of glucose. This tends to confirm that the nervous system requires a continuous supply of glucose in order to function efficiently.

Although the weight of an adult brain is only 2 per cent of the total body weight, the activity of the brain, in terms of utilization of glucose, may amount to 20·5 per cent of the total body activity. In spite of this, the total amount of glucose concentrated within the brain, at any one time, would under normal conditions, be exhausted in 10 to 15 minutes. The actual effects of glucose starvation on the brain and nerve tissue are as follows:

1. Insufficient oxygen.

2. Reduction in specific substances within the brain that are essential for nervous activity.

Circulatory Changes

Not surprisingly the system first affected by a drop in the blood sugar level is the circulatory system. This, of course, includes the heart and blood vessels. When the blood sugar drops, the body automatically reacts in an attempt to restore balance to the system. The main changes that occur involve the adrenal gland, part of which is concerned with the body's reaction to stress situations. This means that if a person has persistent low blood sugar, he may have symptoms similar to those produced by chronic stress. These can include:

1. An irregular increase in the heart rate causing palpitations and breathing difficulties.

2. Angina-like symptoms involving reduction in circulation to the heart muscle, chest cramp and pain in the chest and arms.

3. A general withdrawal of blood to deal with the 'stress effects', causing coldness of the hands and feet, muscular cramp and a poor adaptation to temperature changes.

Glandular Changes

The changes involved in the glandular system following a

drop in the blood glucose level are widespread and could well provide sufficient material for another book. It may, however, be of interest simply to list the glands affected, to emphasize the wide influence of blood sugar imbalance.

1. Pituitary gland. This is the master control gland influencing the thyroid and adrenal glands.

2. Adrenal glands. These glands produce adrenalin and cortisone. It is the persistent stimulation of these glands in a patient suffering from hypoglycaemia that provides the link between hypoglycaemia and rheumatoid arthritis, as overactivity of part of the adrenal glands can cause reduction in the availability of cortisone which gives some protection against joint injury and inflammation.

3. Thyroid gland. Changes that occur with thyroid activity are of less significance than other glands although, like the adrenal and pituitary glands, the thyroid secretions are essentially antagonistic to insulin, and thyroid imbalance may contribute to a blood sugar imbalance.

Digestive Changes

The changes in gastric (stomach) activity are mainly due to the increased insulin level in the blood that occurs with hypoglycaemia rather than the actual deficiency of glucose. A standard hospital test to assess the efficiency of digestive activity is to administer to the patient an injection of insulin. This prompts a rapid and predictable increase in the amount of stomach acids which are then measured. It follows that if this test has such an effect, the fluctuations of the insulin level in the blood, as in hypoglycaemia, would have a similar effect. Indeed, in practice, I find that many patients suffering from stomach ulcers, heartburn, hiatus hernia and other digestive ailments, very often have an underlying blood sugar imbalance.

Many patients with food allergies experience symptoms that may in part be caused by low blood sugar. Unfortunately, the two conditions are often confused, and Chapter 9 deals with this in greater depth.

Patients with coeliac disease, sometimes called non-tropical sprue (gluten intolerance) show very similar symptoms to the flat glucose tolerance curve result seen in some patients with low blood sugar.[1]

Psychological Changes

After discussing the effects of low blood sugar on the brain and nervous system it is not surprising to learn that a patient suffering from hypoglycaemia may also have personality problems. The most common symptoms involving the low blood sugar patient are depression, anxiety and mental confusion. Many researchers, particularly in the United States, consider that hypoglycaemia is the main contributing factor to such serious personality problems as schizophrenia and paranoia. We know that hypoglycaemia affects the adrenal glands and that the adrenal glands are the body's main defence mechanism against stress. It therefore seems likely that the hypoglycaemic patient becomes involved in a vicious circle of adrenal exhaustion causing anxiety and the anxiety causing further exhaustion and stress. Unfortunately, most people suffering from stress tend to overeat, or eat all the wrong foods or miss meals altogether, thus aggravating further the blood sugar imbalance.

Miscellaneous Effects

It is an interesting fact that diabetic patients rarely have asthma. In fact, there are very few cases on record of a true asthma patient having diabetes; the main exception is the condition known as cardiac asthma. Many asthma patients find to their delight in their late 40s and 50s that their asthma symptoms subside. The reason for this is that they often become pre-diabetic; their blood sugar has become raised above normal level thus protecting them from asthma.

The key to this enigma is a substance called histamine. This substance is naturally present in the body and has a variety of uses, not least is its role in controlling osmosis (passage of water) between the body membranes. It is well known that, if the histamine level increases, the character-istic symptoms are hay fever, skin rashes and asthma. The link between histamine and the blood sugar is that histamine and glucose are on separate ends of a see-saw. If the glucose level drops the histamine level rises and vice versa. It follows that a patient who has low blood sugar may, under certain conditions, also have asthma or hay fever and, indeed, many hypoglycaemic patients have children with hay fever. It should be said that low blood sugar is not the *only* cause of asthma; there are certain types of asthma due entirely to stress or extreme sensitivity to various allergens.

The other system of the body affected by hypoglycaemia is the musculo-skeletal system, in other words, muscles and joints. As already explained, the effect of the adrenal glands and, in particular, cortisone on joint inflammation is well documented, hence the apparently miraculous symptom relief afforded to rheumatoid arthritis patients when corti-sone is taken or injected. If the adrenal glands' efficiency is overworked or impaired owing to prolonged low blood sugar, it seems entirely possible that the hypoglycaemic patient would be prone to arthritis and similar problems.

2

THE HYPOGLYCAEMIC PERSONALITY

It is customary to attribute the growth and development of personality to a combination of inherited tendencies and environmental influences. The 'inheritance' school maintain that personality and intelligence are shaped by the genetically laid down characteristics of race and body-type, our personality being determined at birth by these influences. The 'environmental' school believe that we are virtually born with a blank mind which is influenced and moulded in terms of personality and intelligence by our environment. These environmental influences include social class, education, economic considerations, domestic pressures, occupation and health.

Although the controversy over these two fundamental causes of personality has dominated much of the thinking of psychologists, educationists and other workers, recent attitudes support the more balanced view that personality and intelligence are shaped by a combination of both influences.

Leaving aside for the present the question of intelligence, most of us have a many-faceted personality. Our education, parental guidance, choice of partner, employment and religion are all likely to act on our moods, attitudes and beliefs to make us the people we are. A popularly held view is that our adult personality, as presented to the world, is unchanging and unchangeable. We recognize and accept that some people are bad-tempered, moody or depressed, while others are gentle, care-free and optimistic. If someone we know is always angry and aggressive, we usually accept that 'this is the way he is'.

Physical Symptoms and Personality

Many destructive or negative emotions and attitudes are linked with physical symptoms, e.g. depression with fatigue, fear with palpitations and coldness. Physical illnesses associated with stressful attitudes or emotions are often termed 'psychosomatic disorders' or simply 'mind and body illness'. The medical view is that stress produces a physical effect and the treatment of such a disorder needs to be directed at alleviating or masking the stress. This is attempted by prescribing a variety of drugs or by the use of various psychotherapeutic procedures, e.g. psycho-analysis.

The psychologist William James noted in the last century that every emotion has its physical counterpart. This observation appears to support the view that stress affects the physical body, and only by removing the stress can the physical symptom be relieved (i.e. stress-induced stomach ulcers, stress-induced eczema). However, this sequence of cause and effect can be reversed according to the 'chicken and egg principle' – which comes first, the faulty emotion behind the stress, or the physical symptom accompanying the stress?

In practice I have observed that the majority of stressful personalities have accompanying physical symptoms. These physical symptoms often *precede* the emotional changes, e.g. depression preceded by fatigue; anxiety preceded by headache, palpitations and dizziness; agoraphobia preceded by feelings of panic; suicidal tendencies preceded by menstrual disorders and exhaustion.

As explained in the previous chapter, optimum nutrition to the nervous system is a prerequisite of normal health. If the supply of glucose to the nerve cells is deficient, physical symptoms and actual personality changes may occur. The personality of the person suffering from low blood sugar can alter to such an extent that, to all intents and purposes, he or she becomes a different person. Moreover, patients with hypoglycaemia tend to share the same personality patterns.

Before examining the available evidence to support the concept of a hypoglycaemic personality, it may be of value to define more fully the characteristics of a typical hypoglycaemia sufferer, and appreciate the difficulties in diagnosing hypoglycaemia without laboratory evidence.

Difficulties of Diagnosis

The level of glucose in our blood is constantly fluctuating, for demands are made on available glucose when exercising, under stress, during pregnancy and prior to menstruation. In each case there is a tendency for the glucose level to reduce whilst, not surprisingly, our food and drink has the opposite effect of increasing the glucose level. Even the time of day may be significant as the glucose level reduces between meals and at night, or whenever food is avoided for more than three hours.

Diabetic patients on insulin are only too well aware of the sensitive nature of glucose balance as they are obliged to control and monitor constantly their activities and food, as well as their insulin requirements. Most of us, however, are blissfully unaware of the importance of the blood glucose level and the dramatic symptoms that can develop when the level is reduced.

The lowering of blood glucose and the subsequent reduction in available glucose to the nervous system leads to a variety of symptoms as already outlined. Unfortunately for the patient and the diagnostician, the symptoms are neither constant nor predictable, as the available glucose varies to such an extent that sudden and severe physical and emotional symptoms can develop within 15 to 20 minutes following a drop in the glucose level. When the glucose level normalizes ('normal' being the optimum level for that patient) the changes in mood, sudden coldness, palpitations, sweating and many other symptoms attributed to hypoglycaemia, rapidly recede. These sudden shifts in mood and symptoms are often diagnosed as stress-induced. In other words, the patient seeing his doctor with the typical symptoms of low blood sugar is often classified as a neurotic, anxious personality. Regrettably such a diagnosis, with the possible prescription of antidepressants or sedatives, only creates more confusion and worry for the patient. This additional worry can lead to a further imbalance in the blood sugar level and produce an aggravation of the hypoglycaemic symptoms. Hence a vicious circle is achieved.

This train of events is not always so straightforward as Figure 1 suggests, for there is often genuine stress in addition to the hypoglycaemia due to other causes, and this obviously complicates the picture. The fact remains, however, that hypoglycaemia alone can cause the symptoms of stress and a hypoglycaemic personality is very vulnerable to additional stress, often being quite unable to deal with even day-to-day problems. The anxiety created in the patient's mind by a diagnosis of 'nerves' is more damaging if the patient knows full well that he is not under stress and indeed has nothing to

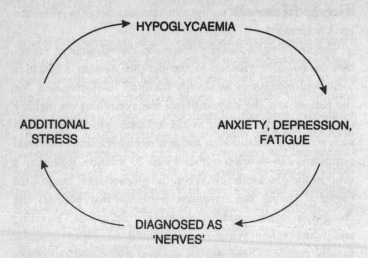

Figure 1 Diagram showing the relation between hypoglycaemia and stress.

worry about. I often hear the comment from patients that they cannot understand why they feel so tense and anxious as they have a settled and happy life with no worries. The medical explanation for anxiety without cause is to suggest that the symptoms, in some strange way, arise from within the patient. This is termed 'endogenous' and is treated as a psychiatric problem with psychotherapy or drugs. It is of great relief to the patient who feels he is 'going mad', or states that he is 'unable to cope anymore', to be told that there is not a nervous breakdown round the corner, nor is his personality breaking up owing to some hidden subconscious mental conflict. What is happening is probably due to an imbalance in his metabolism involving an insufficient supply of fuel to the nervous system (i.e. low blood sugar) which in the majority of cases is easy to treat and often completely reversible.

The Evidence[69]

Having stated that an apparently simple commonplace occurrence involving a drop in the blood glucose level can give rise to profound and sudden physical and emotional symptoms, I feel obliged to justify my comments with a little supportive evidence. Researchers in many countries have, over the last fifty years, examined the problem of hypoglycaemia and the conclusions fall into two distinctly opposing camps. There are those who state that a certain type of personality may give rise to hypoglycaemia, whilst others maintain that hypoglycaemia produces a typical, well-defined personality. The evidence in favour of the latter view is, however, overwhelming. Especially when one appreciates that hypoglycaemia resulting from stomach surgery or insulin therapy can also give rise to the characteristic hypoglycaemic personality.

In the early 1920s Dr Banting and his co-workers (the discoverers of insulin) observed that hypoglycaemia caused by insulin overdose produced symptoms of hunger, weakness and anxiety. These unpleasant symptoms, with which diabetics are usually familiar, are not produced by the insulin itself but by the sudden slump in the level of glucose in the blood, termed a 'hypo' effects. In 1933 two American physicians, Graham and Womack, stated that, 'It is important to emphasize that in many cases the neurological and psychiatric aspects of the condition are so prominent that many of the patients with chronic hypoglycaemia have been referred primarily to neurologists and psychiatrists for treatment.'[2]

Seale Harris, acknowledged as the discoverer of hypoglycaemia, also noted that patients with hypoglycaemia symptoms are often misdiagnosed as neurotic or psychiatric cases. He considered that emotional symptoms can be caused by organic malfunction and reported that dietary treatment resulted in the relief of the symptoms.[3]

Fabrykant, an authority on hypoglycaemia, stated in 1953 that 'personality disorders were secondary to biochemical changes'.[4] In a detailed examination of hypoglycaemia and personality Dr Anthony and his co-workers concluded that their results supported the association of hypoglycaemia with personality disorders. They found that 27 from 31 selected hypoglycaemia patients showed abnormal personality profiles when subjected to standardized psychological testing. Furthermore, three of the remaining four patients were borderline. Their conclusions were summarized as follows:

1. Patients with hypoglycaemia of varying aetiology (diabetic, alimentary or idiopathic) all show the same personality pattern suggesting that hypoglycaemia causes personality disorder.

2. Low blood glucose values with counter-regulatory endocrine reactions constitute a plausible organic explanation for the peculiar mental symptoms that trouble these patients. Our data indicate that reactive hypoglycaemia is almost invariably accompanied by significant personality disorder.[5]

The *British Medical Journal*, 20 April, 1974, carried an article which stated, 'The finding that patients with hypoglycaemia of varying aetiology showed the same personality pattern supports the view that hypoglycaemia causes the abnormality of personality.'[6]

In hypoglycaemia the nervous system is deprived of essential fuel (i.e. glucose) and the brain is subsequently affected. Changes of mood, depression, anxiety, irritability, poor concentration, feelings of panic and suicidal tendencies are just a few of the symptoms that can be produced by this so often misdiagnosed problem. Recent research in the US suggests that even psychiatric and schizoid tendencies may, in part, be due to low blood sugar.

Two researchers, Dr W. Beebe and Dr O. Wendell, wrote in a paper on psychiatric patients that, 'Of those patients categorized as chronic schizophrenics 70 per cent exhibited some form of hypoglycaemia.'[7]

Dr R. Meiers wrote in his paper 'Relative Hypoglycaemia in Schizophrenia', 'Relative Hypoglycaemia is present in up to 70 per cent of patients with schizophrenia. Inadequate diet exists in almost 100 per cent. Since the diet used in the treatment of relative hypoglycaemia also improved nutrition in general, it is a valuable adjunct in the treatment of all patients with schizophrenia.'[8]

Throughout the book I will provide case histories to illustrate the hypoglycaemic personality and, I hope to show the link between physical cause and emotional effect. Hypoglycaemia is not the only cause of disordered personalities, yet it may well be the commonest *physical* cause and certainly the most frequently misdiagnosed.

3

DISCOVERY AND CAUSES

Discovery

Medical discoveries are often made by chance rather than by painstaking research and analysis. One open door may lead to others, for much in nature and science is connected. One clue leads to another, like a treasure trail, and one proven hypothesis may open up a whole field of related study. In this way, the chance observations of an obscure American doctor more than half a century ago led to the discovery that reactive hypoglycaemia is an important cause of a great variety of symptoms. Seale Harris was a general practitioner living in the state of Alabama and a contemporary of Banting and Best, the co-discoverers of the role of insulin in diabetes.

Harris noticed that many diabetic patients attending the new insulin clinics developed symptoms of *low* blood sugar. This paradox is not difficult to understand if you see insulin and sugar as being on opposite ends of the scale. When there is balance the scale is level, but if one is in excess, the other is deficient. Many diabetics have difficulty in accurately judging their insulin requirements and often overdose themselves, producing a condition known as hyperinsulinism which consequently causes hypoglycaemia. This 'hypo' or insulin effect is characterized by symptoms of anxiety, fatigue, breathlessness and palpitations. Essentially the diabetic has swung from high to low blood sugar due to an inappropriate increase in the blood insulin level. Fortunately, this is a transient effect. Most diabetics learn to avoid the 'hypo' situation by carefully balancing their insulin dosage, diet and energy output; at the same time regularly monitoring their blood and urine sugar levels.

To return to Dr Harris, he noted that he had in his practice several patients who exhibited symptoms of the 'hypo' reaction on a regular basis, but who were *not* diabetic and who were, therefore, not taking insulin. He accurately concluded that these patients probably experienced the unpleasant symptoms of hypoglycaemia as a result of overactivity or imbalance in their sugar-regulating apparatus. This complex mechanism involves the islet gland of the pancreas, the liver, to some extent the pituitary, thyroid and adrenal glands and many other factors which play their part in sugar metabolism.

In 1924 Seale Harris presented his theories in a paper published in the *Journal of the American Medical Association*.[9] His reasoning on the possible causes of hypoglycaemia in non-diabetic patients led him to conclude that many glands of the body can be 'hypo' or 'hyper' active and that frequently underactivity (hypo) is preceded by overactivity (hyper). This concept is not difficult to appreciate as overactivity, with subsequent exhaustion or damage, is a characteristic of many organs and systems within the body. Any overworked machine usually malfunctions.

Dr Harris discussed his ideas with Dr Banting who agreed that the role of insulin in hypoglycaemia offered a new aspect to the study of blood sugar balance, presenting a mirror image to the diabetic situation. No papers on this topic had appeared in medical literature prior to Seale Harris's historic work, but his discoveries led to a glut of similar papers in journals all over the world.

The American *Annals of Internal Medicine* (1936) included a further paper by Harris.[3] This definitive statement precisely classified the causes and symptoms of hypoglycaemia. Although subsequent research has shown that the relationship of low blood sugar to excess insulin in the blood is not so simplistic as defined by Harris, it is now recognized that the whole glandular system is involved in the blood sugar balance.

Causes

Having outlined the events that led to the discovery of reactive hypoglycaemia, it is important to discuss the main groups of causes.

1. *Delayed insulin secretion*. Delay, as in early diabetes, causes an inappropriate elevation of insulin at a time when blood glucose is falling.

2. *Alimentary or surgical*. Symptoms known as the 'dumping syndrome' — this involves a rapid emptying of the stomach contents allowing rapid absorption of glucose and resulting reactive hypoglycaemia. This can occur anything from one to four hours after eating.

3. *Nervous factors*. Possible vagal overactivity and stress situations leading to adrenal exhaustion and thyrotoxicosis, etc.

4. *Insulin antagonists*. Suppression of secretion of contra-insulin agents, chiefly growth hormone, adrenal and

pituitary secretions. Treatment by cortisol and growth hormone bring about rapid improvement.

5. *The unknown 90 per cent*. These are mainly thought to be idiopathic, hereditary and largely nutritional in origin, the chief influence being an inherited characteristic coupled with a high starch diet; this gradually gives rise to excessive insulin production.

Perhaps in the fifth cause mentioned the word 'unknown' should be in inverted commas as in my own practice I find that the majority of patients suffering from reactive hypoglycaemia have a characteristic pattern of inherited influences and faulty diet. The typical hypoglycaemic make-up will be discussed in the chapter on diagnosis, for this book is mainly concerned with reactive hypoglycaemia caused by the 'unknown 90 per cent'. I should explain that the medical establishment is not in agreement with the concept of low blood sugar as a 'disease entity' (a condition producing symptoms). Hypoglycaemia is generally seen as a common symptom associated with many disorders. Yet, according to many American nutritionists and non-medical practitioners in Europe, reactive hypoglycaemia is recognized as a condition produced by a variety of causes and giving rise to a large range of clearly-defined symptoms. This is usually caused by the combinations of influences detailed below. It may seem rather illogical to deal with causes after discussing symptoms in Chapter 1, but I believe readers can relate more immediately to symptoms than to causes.

Hereditary Factors

Although we all recognize that characteristics pass through generations, e.g. posture, personality, poor teeth, premature baldness, chest and heart problems, etc., there are, in fact, very few inherited diseases. The list includes syphilis, diabetes and haemophilia. Although other diseases that are directly inherited are more obscure and include certain rare blood disorders and musculo-skeletal problems (chorea and ataxia, etc.) there are, however, many conditions that can be traced through families that have a common theme, i.e. blood sugar imbalance.

If you refer to the list of symptoms of hypoglycaemia in Chapter 1 you will note the following conditions that often run through several generations of the same family – diabetes, epilepsy, asthma, hay fever, migraine, depression, obesity, rheumatoid arthritis. The diabetic patient may produce a diabetic child as the pancreatic deficiency is directly inherited. Paradoxically, the child of a diabetic patient may be born with a normal pancreas that is simply oversensitive rather than deficient and this sensitivity may lead to an eventual over-activity as a result of faulty diet which, in turn, may lead to hyperinsulinism and reactive hypoglycaemia. In my own prac- tice we always enquire about family health, of parents and grandparents and of children and grandchildren.

Table 1 shows the characteristic low blood sugar conditions that run through families. Patients are always asked for details of family health including diabetes, asthma, hay fever and migraine. The list is composed of fifty patients selected from my practice who were diagnosed as hypoglycaemic. They were chosen in strict sequence to avoid giving a biased result.

Organic and Reactive Hypoglycaemia

Some American doctors who specialize in the diagnosis and treatment of hypoglycaemia maintain that we all suffer from the symptoms of hypoglycaemia at some time in our lives.

Some of us, however, are more sensitive to sugar than others. It should be stated that the Western diet contributes to hypoglycaemia owing to the refining, concentrating and high pressure marketing of starch and sugar products.

There are many different causes for hypoglycaemia, including pancreatic tumours, pancreatitis, gastric surgery, adrenal tumours, glandular diseases, etc. However, I am discussing the commonest type of hypoglycaemia known as reactive hypoglycaemia (also called functional hypoglycaemia and relative hypoglycaemia).

The main difference between organic hypoglycaemia and reactive hypoglycaemia lies in the fasting glucose levels. Where there is organic disease causing hypoglycaemia, the glucose fasting level is invariably low. In reactive hypoglycaemia the fasting level of glucose may be normal or even a little above normal, and the body over-reacts to glucose by producing an excess of insulin which creates the drop in blood glucose. In organic hypoglycaemia due to functional disease the symptoms are usually continuous, while in reactive hypoglycaemia the symptoms fluctuate according to type of food, time of day, etc. An inappropriate and unnecessary high sugar diet causes a situation where the blood is flooded with glucose it cannot use. Although some may be stored as glycogen and deposited in the liver or muscles, the balance leads to an over-reaction by the insulin apparatus. In this way the body is conditioned over a period of years to produce more and more insulin until the time is reached where the slightest increase in blood glucose causes a sudden and dramatic increase in the blood insulin.

The final link in this chain of events is the role of the adrenal glands. As the blood sugar drops, the glands produce adrenalin and cortisone to facilitate the release of stored glucose. In this way, further stress symptoms – so characteristic of hypoglycaemia – are produced and the circle starts again.

Patient's condition	Grandparents	Mother	Father	Children	Siblings
M		D			
M		H			
St		A			
M	D				
M	A				A
H & F		M	D		A
M			M		
M		A & M			A
M					HF
F					A
O		D	A		
F		M		A	
F		M	D		M
F		M			
M				M	A
A	A				
B				A	M
M		M			M
M		M	A		
F					A
St	D				
M		A			
O		M			A
M		M	A		
M					A
H		D	M	M	
F		D			
M			D		
M		M			M
B	M				

Patient's condition	Grandparents	Mother	Father	Children	Siblings
M		M	M		M
De		M			
H	M				E
F	D		H		
M		M			
M		M			A
A					A
M			H		
H					A
E					A
M	D				
De			De		HF
De					
HF					HF
M				HF	A
E					M
M			A		
De		M		HF	M
M	A	M		M	
F	A	M			

Key

A	Asthma	H	Headaches
B	Blackouts or dizziness	HF	Hay fever
D	Diabetes	M	Migraine
De	Depression or anxiety	O	Obesity
E	Epilepsy	St	Stomach disorders
F	Fatigue		

Table 1 Chart Showing Hypoglycaemic Conditions in the Families of 50 Patients with Reactive Hypoglycaemia

It has been said that the hypoglycaemia patient of today is the diabetic of tomorrow. As we are talking about totally opposite conditions, this may be at first difficult to understand. Hypoglycaemia, as we know, is characterized by a conditioned over-reaction of the insulin production causing low blood sugar. If, at around sixty years old, the patient's overworked pancreas finally gives up and becomes exhausted, the pendulum swings the other way and the production of insulin is insufficient, thus leading to diabetes.

The diets for hypoglycaemia and diabetes are remarkably similar. The low blood sugar patient avoids sugar to allow the pancreas to reduce and normalize insulin output, while the diabetic needs to avoid sugar because his body does not produce enough insulin to convert, transport and utlilize the sugar. In many glandular imbalances, whether affecting thyroid, pituitary or adrenal glands, the line between overactivity and underactivity may be very finely drawn, as an imbalance can occur either way, but in the early stages the problem can often be reversed if correct treatment is applied.

4

SUGAR:
AN UNNATURAL
HISTORY

To most people sugar is the white or brown substance with which they sweeten tea or coffee. This is known as sucrose and is extracted from beet or cane. The other main sugars consumed are lactose (milk sugar) and fructose (fruit sugar). The whole sugar family, known as carbohydrates, is shown in Table 2. They are classified according to their complexity, the simple sugars being monosaccharides and the most complex sugars are polysaccharides consisting of many groups of simple units.

In studies it has been found that the average adult carbohydrate consumption can be broken down as follows:

Starch (bread, cereals, etc.)	50%
Sucrose (sugar)	35%
Lactose (milk, etc.)	7%
Glucose and fructose (fruit and vegetables)	8%

Early Use of Sugar

The general use of sugar probably began around 1000BC in

the later Bronze Age, the main source of sweetening for cereals and cooking being honey. At first wild bees' nests were ransacked but, with the spread of pastureland, crude beekeeping leading to hive manufacturing took place. The production of honey in the Bronze Age was secondary to the need for beeswax, an essential substance in the process of bronze casting. Understandably, people learned to enjoy the sweet flavour of the honey for it served as a seasoning as well as a sweetener. Although sugar was extracted from sugar cane in India several centuries before Christ, honey remained the main sweetener, sugar being used chiefly as a medicine.

The Romans used honey exclusively in their cooking and by Anglo-Saxon times honey was still the sweetening agent for food and drink. The production of honey became an essential part of country life, and laws controlling and taxing the ownership of hives were introduced.

After the Dark Ages following the fall of Rome, it was the Crusaders of the eleventh century who rediscovered honey in Europe. Also, the gradual spread of sugar cane production from India to Persia had been accelerated by the Arab conquests. As a result, cane was grown in North Africa and the Mediterranean isles by the tenth century. With the impetus of the Crusades, trade flourished between the Eastern Mediterranean and Europe and sugar became one of the most sought-after commodities.

Sugar at this time was very expensive, being rare and costly to import. It was only available to the very rich, and honey, being cheaper, was still the only sweetener for the poor. In medieval England sugar was regarded as a spice or flavouring, being used to flavour both sweet and savoury dishes. In the homes of the rich merchants and noblemen, even meat was dusted with sugar. It was also used as a medicine for a variety of ailments, particularly for convalescence and infections.

World Scale Production

With the colonizing of the many islands of the Americas in the fifteenth and sixteenth centuries, sugar cane was the ideal economic crop and was grown on an increasing scale. Barbados, Trinidad and Jamaica became part of the British Empire, while the Portuguese controlled the Azores, and the Spanish colonized the Canaries, Cuba and Puerto Rico. This led to an increase in the world production and consumption of sugar, and in the late sixteenth century there were 50 refineries in London alone.

In spite of the then heavy taxation on sugar importation, demand grew. In the reign of Elizabeth I, the consumption was 1lb (450g) per person per year but, with the price equivalent in the twentieth century prices of around £20 per lb, only the very wealthy could afford its regular use. Within a hundred years consumption rose to 4lb (1.8kg) per person and even the poorest folk bought a few ounces a week. It was still considered a good medicine and many prescriptions included sugar to purge the 'vapours' or 'melancholy'. The damaging effects of sugar were, however, beginning to be apparent: Elizabeth I had black teeth owing to her sugar craving.

Sugar consumption took a great surge upwards with the introduction of tea, coffee and chocolate in the eighteenth century. All these drinks are naturally slightly bitter, and tea with sugar became a favourite drink of the poor. By the late eighteenth century, sugar and tea were staple items in the inadequate diet of the poor in the industrial towns of England.

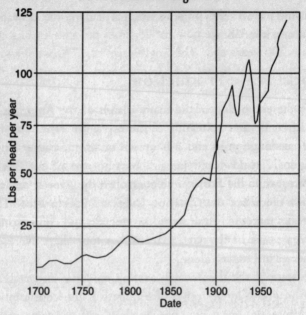

Figure 2 Sugar consumption in Britain

Present Consumption

This brings the story almost up to date, and the consumption of sugar has grown enormously in the last 150 years (see Figure 2).

As can be seen, we now eat 120lb (54kg) per year each. Obviously, some eat more than others, yet most people, being confronted with these figures, will stoutly deny that they eat anywhere near the average of 2½lb (1kg) sugar a week. Much of the sugar we eat is not visible sugar: many items of food and drink contain sugar as a sweetener or preservative, and this 'hidden' sugar is included in the consumption figures. Table 3 gives some idea of the amount of 'hidden' sugar in typical foods.

The world production of sugar has grown from 1½ million

tons in 1850 to the present level of 75 million tons per annum. In the UK we now eat 25 times the amount of sugar we ate 200 years ago. The Englishman of 1780 would have taken two years to eat the same amount of sugar his 1980 counterpart eats in one month.

The intake of sugar is not spread evenly over the population, as it has been shown that there is a disproportionately high consumption in young people, the highest consumption being in 12 to 14 year olds. Children in general eat twice as much sugar and starch as the national average, and consumption in the UK is currently the highest in the world. This depressing picture indicates that the average child in this country obtains between 25 and 35 per cent of his/her total calories from sugar.

Why All the Fuss?

Professor John Yudkin in his book *Pure, White and Deadly* makes two very significant statements which are worth quoting. First, '. . . there is no physiological requirement for sugar', and second, '. . . if only a small fraction of what is already known about the facts of sugar were to be revealed in relation to any other material used as a food additive, the material would promptly be banned'.[10]

How has the confusion over sugar arisen? To most people it is a necessary source of energy and we are told 'it helps us work, rest and play'. Glucose drinks are given to aid convalescence, barley sugar and chocolate are prescribed for fatigue and glucose tablets recommended for sportsmen. The confusion arises perhaps from the use of the word 'sugar' for, as I have already shown, there are many sugars. Sugar as glucose *is* needed as an essential fuel for the body, especially the nervous system, but we do not need to *eat* glucose. The

Table 2 Classification of carbohydrates (simplified)	
Mono-saccharides	basic unit
Di-saccharides	2 mono-saccharide units
Poly-saccharides	10-10,000 mono-saccharide units

Mono-saccharides (single sugars)

Glucose (dextrose): Found in blood, oxidized in cells to provide energy. Stored in the liver as glycogen.

Fructose (fruit sugar): Found in fruit and honey – sweetest of the sugars.

Galactose: Obtained from milk sugar, not found free in nature.

Di-saccharides (double sugars)

Sucrose (cane or beet sugar): Not directly absorbed by blood stream, except after splitting by digestive enzymes in small intestine into the two single sugars glucose and fructose, which are then separately absorbed or converted to glycogen.

Maltose (Malt sugar): Present in barley and in honey, though occurs chiefly as a result of starch breakdown by saliva and by secretions from the pancreas. Like sucrose it must be split by enzymes in the small intestine into glucose units before it can be used.

Lactose (milk sugar): Like the other di-saccharides, lactose cannot be utilized by the body until broken down by digestive enzymes into the two single sugars, glucose and galactose. In some infants a 'block' may exist whereby the galactose cannot be absorbed and the child will become ill, even fatally, unless milk is withheld.

Poly-saccharides

Examples are starch, dextrins, cellulose and glycogen. The polysaccharides are made up of simple glucose units bonded together and cannot be utilized by the body until 'uncoupled' by digestive processes. They are insoluble in cold water, but cooking softens and ruptures cells and facilitates digestion.

Table 3 Sugar content of food

Food	Amount	Sugar equivalent in teaspoonful
Chocolate fudge	4 oz (100g)	14
Chewing gum	1 stick	3
Chocolate cake	1 medium slice	14
Sponge cake	1 medium slice	6
Doughnut	Small	4
Average biscuit	1 biscuit	2
Baked custard	½ cupful	4
Ice cream	5 oz (150g)	6
Apple pie	1 medium slice	12
Chocolate sauce	1 teaspoonful	4
Jam	1 tablespoonful	3
Honey	1 tablespoonful	3
Cocoa (all milk)	1 cupful	5
Coca-Cola	1 bottle	4

glucose should enter our bodies as an integral part of various unrefined and complex foods, gradually being broken down in a step by step process before passing into the blood as glucose. It may also be made available, if required, by the conversion of glycogen stored in the liver. In this way, the available glucose is utilized for energy as required, or stored if not required. Eating large amounts of glucose (as sugar, etc.) bypasses the normal digestive step ladder and presents the body with a substance it simply cannot fully utilize. In a natural environment, we can obtain sugar only by eating unrefined cereals or fruit, and our normal appetite would not allow us to eat more than a limited amount. This would be digested and the glucose gradually released.

The refining of starch has led to a situation where we can eat large amounts of concentrated sugar. Unfortunately, the human digestive system has yet to adapt to the changes in our dietary habits. As a result, the modern diet is very different from the ideal diet for man that has evolved over millions of years.

One important factor that allows for the high consumption of sugar, is its cheapness. In the sixteenth century the cost of sugar was equivalent to the present cost of caviar, and, in fact, its price has fallen to only 0.5 per cent of the fifteenth century price. In spite of this, the income from the sale of sugar and confectionery in the UK is at present around £2,000 million per year.

Dead Calories

Sugar is either eaten in addition to a normal diet or it replaces the more valuable foods in the diet. Approximately 500 calories a day are supplied by sugar in the typical British diet. It follows that sugar eaters will either (a) put on weight, or (b) be deprived of food that is replaced by sugar.

It is not the brief of this book to detail the harmful effects of sugar but, as hypoglycaemic patients have a craving for sugar, they are usually prone to the effects of a high sugar diet. The damaging effects of sugar are well reviewed in many publications.[10 27 56]

5

MIGRAINE

Symptoms

Someone once wrote, 'There are headaches and there are migraine headaches.' It is perhaps wrong to classify migraine as a headache, although the word 'migraine' implies hemicranial or half-head. It should be stated, before going further, that a headache is never the only symptom experienced during a migraine attack. The complete syndrome, sometimes termed 'common migraine', involves various components grouped as follows.

HEADACHE

Usually one-sided but may be both sides of the head. Great variations exist in severity and duration, but rarely less than two to three hours and can last seven to ten days. (I have encountered patients who have awakened with a headache every morning.) Intensity can vary enormously from a constant dull ache to an incapacitating, throbbing and violent pain. Pain may be above the eyes, at the base of the skull or may occasionally travel to the face and jaw, producing symptoms similar to trigeminal neuralgia.

NAUSEA

Migraine is often referred to as a sick headache, for nausea often accompanies the headache. There may be a tendency to vomit or a feeling of nausea associated with the smell or even the sight of food. Other symptoms frequently accompany the nausea, including heartburn, over-salivation, hiccup, belching and retching. Sometimes the vomiting signals the end of the migraine. If, however, vomiting is severe, protracted and accompanied by heavy sweating, the resulting fluid depletion may lead to prostration.

APPEARANCE

In severe cases the patient has the look of someone in shock, with pale drawn features. There may be puffiness and oedema of the face, often around one eye or to the side of the mouth. At the onset of a migraine the face may be bright red, suddenly turning pale.

VISUAL SYMPTOMS

A variety of symptoms affect the eyes, the commonest being photophobia (sensitivity to light), blurring of vision or blood-shot eyes.

DIGESTIVE SYMPTOMS

Some migraine sufferers experience cramp-like pains in the stomach, constipation, distension with occasional diarrhoea and sharp colic-type pain as the attack progresses. This effect is sometimes termed 'abdominal migraine'.

SINUS SYMPTOMS

Symptoms similar to hay fever or chronic rhinitis may precede a migraine attack. Nasal stuffiness and loss of smell may be experienced with frequent sneezing.

FATIGUE

A frequent symptom of migraine is a feeling of lethargy and drowsiness with occasional pronounced muscular weakness and heaviness. Insomnia is common, the brief periods of sleep being very deep and dream-filled.

BALANCE

For a variety of reasons migraine sufferers often feel dizzy or faint and may have difficulty in focusing their eyes.

WATER RETENTION

A characteristic of migraine patients is a tendency to retain fluid during an attack. The mechanism of this will be discussed in a later chapter and is due to an imbalance in the sodium/potassium ratio.

EMOTIONAL CHANGES

Not surprisingly, the moods of the person experiencing a migraine attack will vary with the symptoms. There are, however, predictable mood changes that are symptomatic of migraine. These include: initial anxiety followed by depression; severe agitation and fits of bad temper, followed by despair and apathy if the attack is protracted.

OTHER SYMPTOMS

The severity of a migraine attack can lead to some very unusual symptoms, including nose bleeds; hot flushings; extreme sensitivity to noise; and a distortion of certain tastes and smells.

Many migraine attacks are preceded by what is termed an 'aura' or classical migraine. In early medical literature this strange effect was likened to visions or trances and has been recognized as an early warning of migraine for over

2,000 thousand years. The aura may be experienced as a mild hallucination or a dream-like loss of contact with reality. To most sufferers, however, it is simply an awareness that an attack is imminent, yet most migraine patients find it very difficult to explain the exact nature of their 'warning'.

Many different types of migraine have been defined according to their pattern of cause and frequency. It has often been stated that there is no such thing as a typical migraine and those who have never experienced a migraine attack or do not have a migraine sufferer in their immediate family, are sometimes puzzled and unsympathetic about the fuss caused by 'just a headache'. The nearest experience to a migraine attack for many of us is a severe hangover. All the components are there – the sensitive eyes, feeling of sickness, a splitting headache and a tendency to jump at slight noises. These symptoms are usually accompanied by a feeling of mental and physical lethargy and a feeling that it would be preferable if one were allowed to quietly die. On a more serious note, the migraine sufferer and the drunkard are both suffering from an imbalance in their metabolism. For different reasons their blood glucose level has fallen and precipitated the distressing symptoms they are experiencing. Small wonder that the majority of migraine sufferers cannot tolerate alcohol.

The actual cause of a migraine headache at the site (within the brain) is thought to be a localized vasodilation (increased pressure within the blood vessels causing them to swell). This results in pressure, irritation and pain and, as the cranial nerves become affected, problems are referred to the eyes, ears, liver and stomach. To understand the link between this vasodilation and low blood sugar, it is necessary to discuss, step by step, how one affects the other.

Migraine and Blood Sugar

Glucose is almost the only fuel required by nerve tissue and, understandably, the body always gives priority to the supply of fuel to the brain and nervous system. To facilitate this, automatic compensatory reactions take place when the glucose level drops, for, under normal conditions, the total glucose concentration within the brain would be exhausted within 10-15 minutes if glucose were not readily available. (It has been shown that a drop of as little as five per cent in the glucose requirement to the brain creates symptoms of nerve deprivation, i.e. neuroglycopenia.) The glucose supplied to the brain is topped up by an automatic increase in blood volume. In other words, reduced quality leads to increased quantity. In this way, although the concentration of glucose has been reduced, sufficient glucose is made available to brain and nerve tissue by the simple expedient of increasing the flow of blood to the brain. Unfortunately, if this compensatory mechanism operates too frequently on a regular basis, owing to the repeated lowering of the blood glucose level, the nerve tissues become oversensitive from the pressure of the bulging blood vessels passing through them. It is this increased blood-pressure that creates the headache and other symptoms.

In a group of 35 migraine sufferers given a six-hour glucose tolerance test, all 35 were diagnosed as hypoglycaemic.[11] In my practice I have found that, of the migraine patients tested for low blood sugar, 92 per cent were confirmed as hypoglycaemic. It would seem that, although migraine is a complex and distressing problem with many trigger factors, the principal underlying cause is an imbalance in the blood glucose level.

Migraine attacks frequently follow a predictable pattern.

They may occur just before or during menstruation, after eating chocolate, cheese or drinking alcohol. A common trigger is fatigue or stress, and even strenuous exercise can initiate an attack. Many sufferers from migraine and lesser headaches find that the commonest pattern is the headache on wakening. Often the headache will occur at almost exactly the same time each morning. This is not difficult to understand when one realizes that the level of blood sugar drops to its lowest point in the early hours between 3 a.m. and 5 a.m.[62] By the same token, the asthma sufferer becomes wheezy and distressed early in the morning, for the same causative factors prevail.

A tendency exists in medical circles to attribute the cause of migraine to a great variety of factors, varying from food allergy and sensitivity to stress and personality problems. There are obviously many different causes of headaches, some trivial, others extremely serious. There seems little doubt, however, that the type of headache known as migraine is, in the vast majority of cases, due to blood sugar imbalance.

Case History

Pauline, a 43-year-old secretary, had suffered migraine attacks over 25 years. The headaches occurred every seven to ten days and lasted approximately 24 hours. They also occurred pre-menstrually for three to four days. Her other symptoms included photophobia (light sensitivity), fatigue, nausea and sugar-cravings (which were worse before periods). Her mother had been a migraine sufferer and her daughter was a hay-fever sufferer.

Pauline's diet was poor, consisting of 12 to 15 cups of tea daily with two spoons of sugar in each. She avoided breakfast since she 'couldn't face food until lunchtime'; then she had a sandwich lunch and dinner at around 6 p.m.

The Hair Mineral Analysis showed low levels of chromium, manganese, magnesium and potassium. The six-hour glucose tolerance test gave a normal fasting level of 4.2mmol/litre which fell rapidly during the test to a low level of 2.2mmol/litre.

Pauline was encouraged to eat regularly and avoid sugar. Supplements were prescribed to improve the mineral status and support the adrenal glands. After initial problems with the diet, she became symptom-free in 16 weeks.

6

ASTHMA AND
HAY FEVER

Asthma was first described 1,800 years ago by Aretaeus the Cappadocian, significantly the same physician who identified the symptoms of diabetes.

Causes of Asthma

Although these two conditions frequently exist in the same family, it is usually assumed that a genetic imbalance in some way splits, producing either diabetes or asthma. In spite of the common occurrence of both conditions in the same family, they never occur together in one person (except in very rare cases which will be discussed later). The common denominator in the asthma patient and the diabetic patient is blood sugar imbalance, the asthmatic having hypoglycaemia and the diabetic having hyperglycaemia. It should be said, however, that not all hypoglycaemics have asthma, nor do all asthmatics have hypoglycaemia. There is a type of asthma known as psychic or 'stress' asthma that has a psychological cause. However, the evidence to support the view that hypoglycaemia is the main cause of asthma is overwhelming. (Between the years 1959 and 1966 the death rate from asthma increased *eight times* among the 10-14 year olds — just the age for highest sugar consumption.)[12]

The medical view that asthma is triggered by an allergen, e.g. pollen or a stress situation, is not supported by the timing of a typical asthma attack. Most asthmatics experience symptoms in the early hours, often being awakened by the distressing symptoms of suffocation and breathlessness. Significantly, the pollen count drops to its lowest level at night and the sufferer cannot be under a great deal of stress when he or she is asleep in bed! The blood sugar level, however, is at its lowest level between 3 a.m. and 5 a.m., hence the onset of symptoms at this time.

If we accept the notion that asthmatics suffer from low blood sugar — where is the evidence? Diabetics are thought to be protected from asthma by their high blood sugar level, for the only condition leading to a person having both asthma and diabetes is that of dysinsulinism. Here the alteration of high and low blood sugar leads to symptoms of both disorders. This rare condition is thought to be due to a delay in insulin production (leading to high blood sugar) followed by an inappropriate excess of insulin (low blood sugar). This imbalance can be identified and diagnosed by the use of a six-hour glucose tolerance test.

It is interesting to note that the drugs commonly used for asthma relief act by raising the blood sugar, e.g. cortisone, adrenalin, etc. Furthermore, the habit of prescribing sugar or glucose injections to stop an asthma attack only serves to alleviate the symptoms for a short time. The resulting rise in blood sugar level is rapidly followed by a drop in the sugar level due to stimulation of the pancreas and the insulin reaction, and the asthma symptoms reappear.

In 1939, Joslyn, a renowned authority on diabetes, drew attention to the 'protective role' of diabetes in relation to asthma. He noted that many asthmatics who develop diabetes rapidly lose their asthma symptoms.[13]

Many glands in the body produce substances that have an antagonistic or opposite effect to insulin. One of these is the thyroid which produces a hormone called thyroxine. As long ago as 1913, asthma was frequently treated by prescribing thyroid extract, as it was found that many asthmatics had underactive thyroids. This reduced secretion of thyroxine led to an oversecretion of insulin, which, in turn, resulted in hypoglycaemia. Conversely, it was observed that patients with overactive or toxic thyroids often lost their asthma symptoms, and removal of the enlarged gland caused a return of the asthma.

The mechanism whereby a decrease in the blood sugar level triggers off the symptoms of asthma (and indeed many other allergies) is not fully understood. The results of recent research work, however, suggest that the substance histamine, which affects cell permeability and tissue fluid balance, is present in abnormal amounts in the blood of allergic persons. Significantly, the stressful, hypoglycaemic patient also has an elevated blood histamine level, possibly due to the over-production of histamine by the body when under stress. Although this is an extremely complex process, it is thought that the breakdown and utilization of protein from body tissue, accelerated under conditions of stress, leads to the release of excess histamine into the blood.

Under normal conditions, the body, in its wisdom, has a safeguard to avoid an excessive build-up of histamine. It releases a substance from the liver known as histaminase which destroys the surplus histamine. If, however, the liver is congested or damaged owing to wrong diet, drug abuse, alcoholism or hepatitis, then this safeguard is weakened or removed and the histamine remains high. (The relationship between liver congestion and the characteristic high starch diet of the hypoglycaemic is well known. The excessive consumption of starch leads to a surplus of glucose which the body converts to glycogen for storage in the liver and other tissues. If, however, the intake of starch is out of proportion to the utilization of glycogen, there is an inevitable build-up in the liver leading to congestion and malfunction.) On the face of it, the taking of antihistamine drugs would seem to be a simple solution to this problem. Many investigators have shown, however, that the use of drugs to reduce the histamine level is not the answer, as the drugs themselves can cause further liver damage because of their toxicity.[14]

Case History

Ken, an 18-year-old student, had suffered asthma since birth. His symptoms were aggravated by stress and sudden weather changes. The attacks of breathlessness were always worse between 3 a.m. and 5 a.m. His grandfather had been an asthmatic and his younger brother was a hay-fever sufferer.

Vega testing failed to show any obvious food or environmental allergy. The Hair Mineral Analysis indicated low levels of magnesium, chromium and zinc. A six-hour glucose tolerance test showed a flat 'fatigue curve', with a low level of 2.5mmol/litre.

Ken's diet was average, but he drank six to eight cups of coffee daily with two spoons of sugar in each; he smoked 12 cigarettes daily and drank approximately 12 to 15 pints of lager each week.

Dietary recommendations were given to balance the blood sugar, avoiding sugar, alcohol and cigarettes. A vitamin B complex and mineral supplements were recommended, with adrenal support formula. Additionally, Ken was prescribed 8gm of vitamin C daily. Osteopathic treatment was also given to improve chest mobility and lung capacity.

After a while Ken was able to reduce his medication to very occasional use, and he remains today virtually symptom free.

However, he continues with 3–4gms of vitamin C daily and follows the hypoglycaemic diet closely.

Hay Fever

Although the symptoms of hay fever are not as serious as asthma, it is nonetheless a distressing condition. Research has shown that the hay fever sufferer also shows a characteristic blood sugar imbalance. As the area affected in hay fever involves the nose, eyes and upper respiratory system, it is inevitable that hay fever is usually triggered off by airborne irritation, e.g. pollen, household dust, etc. Although not so easily affected by food or stress as is asthma, the role of various trigger factors in hay fever can be more significant than in asthma.

In my experience there is a background, low profile hypoglycaemia in most hay fever sufferers, which is expressed in a seasonal sensitivity to dust or pollen. The medically defined condition known as chronic rhinitis or sinusitis can be seen as chronic hay fever. The sufferer experiences stuffed nose and inflamed eyes, particularly in the morning on waking. He cannot tolerate dust of any kind, the irritation from which sets up a whole series of sneezes.

There is a need, therefore, in all the respiratory/allergy problems, to consider the possibility of low blood sugar as the prime cause, irrespective of the types of trigger factors or the diversity of symptoms.

We cannot escape the fact that correct nutrition should be the first consideration in successfully treating these distressing complaints.

Case History
Sara was a music student who suffered from seasonal hay fever

from April to September and recurring allergic rhinitis during the Autumn and Winter. She found these symptoms very distressing, particularly as she was very prone to infections and was rarely without a 'snuffle' or a 'sneeze'. There were many triggers to the onset of symptoms including dusty and smoky atmospheres, fatigue and stress. Symptoms were often worse before her period. Her brother had asthma and her older sister was a migraine sufferer.

The six-hour glucose tolerance test showed a normal fasting level of 4.8mmol/litre with a rapid fall to 2.7mmol/litre during the test. A Hair Mineral Analysis showed low levels of chromium, magnesium and potassium with a very low level of zinc. The Vega test showed a strong response to house dust mites, cigarette smoke and mixed grasses and pollens.

Sara had a sweet tooth and her diet reflected this, consisting of toast and honey for breakfast, crisps and biscuits for lunch and ice-cream or cake after her evening meal. She ate approximately 4ozs of chocolate daily and rarely ate salads or fruit. The low sugar, hypoglycaemic diet was prescribed with supplementary minerals and B vitamins and 4gms of vitamin C daily; extra zinc was also prescribed. In addition, Sara was desensitized on grasses, pollens, cigarette smoke and house dust mites using homoeopathically prepared allergy remedies.

Progress was slow as treatment was started only weeks before the hay fever season, but over the following year symptoms cleared completely.

7

RHEUMATISM AND ARTHRITIS

Rheumatism and arthritis are broad terms to describe a whole family of muscle and joint problems. Arthritis means simply 'inflammation of the joints'. The commonest members of this large family are osteo-arthritis, gout and rheumatoid-arthritis.

Osteo-arthritis can be seen as accelerated wear and tear and, not surprisingly, affects chiefly the weight-bearing joints, e.g. knees and hips, and the joints involved in the most activity, e.g. thumb and wrist.

Gout is essentially an expression of a biochemical imbalance involving a gradual silting up of certain joints by crystals of uric acid. This occurs as a result of an imbalance in the blood leading to a precipitation of excessive uric acid into crystals causing swelling, redness and severe pain. The joints mainly affected are the weight-bearing joints of the lower extremities, especially the great toes and knees. Although the excessive eating of certain proteins and wines is an important factor in gout (being almost an epidemic amongst the wealthy classes in the seventeenth and eighteenth centuries, so much so that special gout stools were available upon which the Regency gentlemen could rest their painful swollen feet), there are, however, other causes of gout apart from nutritional imbalances.

Rheumatoid arthritis is the most widespread and perhaps the least understood of the arthritis family. The characteristic symptoms include fatigue; pain; distortion and swelling of the extremity joints – especially the hands; loss of power in muscles and eventual disablement in many cases. Several theories have been offered to explain the causes of rheumatoid arthritis, ranging from an inherited tendency to stress to the inevitable virus. Current medical thinking, however, suggests that the condition represents a breakdown in the body's immune system, leading to a situation where the sufferer develops antibodies to his own tissues. Instead of the antibodies fighting bacteria or virus they act against the body. This is known as an auto-immune response.

Treatment

A recent popular publication on arthritis and rheumatism lists the treatment for arthritis as follows:[15]

1. Rest

2. Occupational therapy and appliances; adaptations to the home.

3. Splints and plasters.

4. Physiotherapy.

5. Drugs.

6. Surgery.

It is interesting to note that no mention is made of correct nutrition.

Osteo-arthritis is treated mainly with heat, exercise, physiotherapy, drugs and injections and, as a last resort, surgical joint replacement. Very little attention is paid to joint misalignment, tissue health, diet and weight control.

Traditionally, gout was treated by avoidance of the proteins that lead to the uric acid build-up. These include certain fish, liver, sweetbreads, brain and red wine. This 'low purine' diet, unfortunately, only controls and does very little to cure. Modern drug treatment is equally superficial, drugs being prescribed to reduce the formation of uric acid (e.g. allopurinol) and to increase loss of uric acid via the kidneys. For the greater majority of patients suffering from the various joint problems discussed, the treatment is usually analgesics or anti-inflammatory drugs. For many it is a waiting game as the masked symptoms gradually worsen to the point of incapacity or surgery.

Perhaps the most controversial treatment is the use of steroids (cortisone, prednisolone and ACTH) as they are considered by many to be miracle drugs, and by others to be very harmful. It may be worth looking more closely at this particular treatment.

CORTISONE

Cortisone, and hydro-cortisone, are natural substances produced by the cortex of the adrenal glands. Their main role, as explained in Chapter 8, is in carbohydrate metabolism. Since their original discovery as a possible treatment for arthritis in the 1940s, a bewildering range of synthetic materials with similar structure has been produced. Perhaps the best known are prednisone and prednisolone.

ACTH (CORTICOTROPIN)

This substance is not produced by the adrenal glands but is, in fact, released by the anterior pituitary gland in the forehead. This master gland releases various substances that activate or stimulate other glands. (One author described the pituitary gland as 'the conductor of the glandular orchestra'.) The action of ACTH is to stimulate the adrenal cortex. In this roundabout way, cortisone production is also increased. ACTH is considered less harmful than cortisone, for it creates fewer-side effects.

EFFECTS AND SIDE-EFFECTS

As long ago as 1936, the Canadian physiologist Professor Hans Selve noted that large amounts of corticosteroid hormones were produced as part of the body's adaptation to stress.[16] With prolonged stress, there can occur adrenal exhaustion with the inevitable reduction in cortisone flow. It is not fully understood how cortisone affects joints, but we do know it has an important role in protecting joints against inflammation. Hence the dramatic improvement in arthritic patients when they take cortisone. Significantly, most arthritic sufferers have a history of stress which would, of course, deplete their own cortisone level. When cortisone was first used for arthritis, doctors were convinced that if the body produced sufficient cortisone, simply providing additional cortisone would not bring about improvement. Therefore, when cortisone was prescribed for arthritic patients and produced apparently miraculous changes, it was assumed that arthritic patients were deficient in adrenal hormones.

Unfortunately, time has shown that the body does not need extra cortisone, and side-effects — many quite devastating — are caused by regularly taking cortisone and other steroids. A safer and more logical approach is to provide adequate nutrition to meet the demands of stress and, in addition, take substances that we know will increase the body's own cortisone flow. Dr Roger Williams, the discoverer of the B vitamin pantothenic acid, advocates this important vitamin as a treatment for arthritis and gout since, without it, cortisone cannot be produced.[17] Research work has shown that the adrenal glands actually shrivel and the hormone flow is markedly reduced when pantothenic acid is not available.

Arthritis and Low Blood Sugar

You may well comment at this stage, 'Very interesting, but what has this to do with low blood sugar?'

In 1906, Francis Hare, a British psychiatrist, published a massive book on food ecology called *The Food Factor in Disease*. In this he stated that many conditions, including migraine, asthma, eczema, epilepsy, angina, gout and rheumatoid arthritis were caused by the excessive consumption of starch and sugar. This view was based on his observations that patients on such a diet showed dramatic symptom improvement when they reduced their starch and replaced the sugary foods with protein. He also found that patients on high sugar diets were, in fact, addicted to sugar, and severe withdrawal symptoms were noted after reducing their sugar intake for a few days. This malaise and depression would often cause the patient to return to his sugar after which he would feel better.

Medical workers have never been quick to adopt new ideas, and the concept that diet in any way influenced the cause of disease was quite revolutionary. Unfortunately, this notion still pervades present medical attitudes. Although, perhaps, his terminology was slightly different, Dr Hare was anticipating Seale Harris's theories by 30 years. He was, of course, describing exactly the cause, symptoms and withdrawal effects of the typical hypoglycaemic sufferer.

Hormones

It is an interesting fact that many of the conditions attributed to low blood sugar improve during pregnancy. This particularly applies to migraine, epilepsy, gastric ulcers and rheumatoid arthritis. Dr Abrahamson, an American authority in hypoglycaemia, attributes this to '. . . the large amounts of pituitary hormones and cortisone which, being antagonistic to insulin, will tend to allow the glucose level to increase and conditions in which low blood sugar are found will therefore tend to become milder'.[18] I have noticed in my practice that arthritic patients tend to follow the characteristic pattern of low blood sugar sufferers, often improving dramatically during pregnancy but, conversely, experiencing a severe flare-up of symptoms immediately before periods. Although very little work has been carried out to show a link between pre-menstrual tension, arthritis symptoms and low blood sugar, there is an interesting clue to a possible common factor, the mineral calcium.

Calcium

It has been known for over 30 years that low blood sugar is accompanied by a low calcium level in the blood. A characteristic of low blood sugar is, as we know, a tendency to hyperinsulinism with resulting overactivity in the stomach secretions. Unless the gastric acid (pH) is normal, calcium is not absorbed. This can create a situation where rheumatic patients with low blood sugar may be withdrawing calcium from the bones to maintain a normal level of blood calcium.

Another aspect of the role of calcium in hypoglycaemia is that a reduced blood calcium level leads to a hyper-sensitivity and irritability of the nervous system. This can cause muscle cramps and spasm.

Although the body contains more calcium than any other mineral, the absorption of calcium is very inefficient for only 10-30 per cent of the calcium consumed is absorbed. With this in mind, it is worth noting that, under stress, absorption is decreased and excretion increased. (The role of calcium and low blood sugar is expressed in diagram form in Figure 3.)

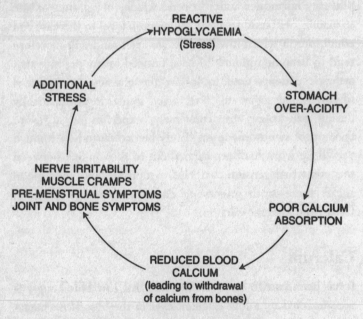

Figure 3 The role of calcium in reactive hypoglycaemia

To summarize, the low level of calcium in the blood of arthritic patients may well be attributed to the low blood sugar and the high insulin found in their blood. Thus a vicious circle is complete, for a calcium deficiency can lead to weak bones, muscle cramps and nerve irritability. This irritability can lead to further stress and resulting hypoglycaemia.

Pre-menstrual Syndrome

Women patients with rheumatoid arthritis invariably feel an aggravation of symptoms prior to and during periods. The calcium level drops steadily and predictably eight or ten days before the period, causing pre-menstrual tension, depression and headache. Dr Roger Williams has listed the symptoms of calcium deficiency as anxiety neurosis, fatigue, insomnia and tension.[17] The system reacts to this situation as it would to stress, producing extra cortisone and, inevitably, fluid retention. The muscle cramps associated with calcium deficiency may affect the emptying womb, causing abdominal pain and spasm.

You will begin to understand why calcium is so often prescribed for low blood sugar, and why rheumatoid arthritis should, in many cases, be seen as yet another condition related to hypoglycaemia.

Case History

Chris, a 33-year-old housewife, had suffered bouts of pre-menstrual syndrome following the birth of her only child five years previously. Her symptoms began nine to ten days before each period and ceased promptly when the period started. Symptoms included irritability, morning fatigue, loss of sex drive, sugar craving, acne and breast tenderness. Her cycle had been 38 days since the onset of these symptoms.

A six-hour glucose tolerance test showed a low fasting level of 3mmol/litre, the lowest point during the test being 2.4mmol/litre. The hair mineral analysis was normal except for a low level of chromium and zinc.

Chris was prescribed an appropriate diet to improve the blood sugar balance and supplementary chromium and zinc. In addition, a B-complex and extra vitamin B_6 were recommended. Because of the link between the adrenal and ovarian activities and blood sugar, she was also given adrenal and ovarian glandulars.

Chris became symptom-free in four months and her cycle normalized at 28 days.

Osteo-arthritis and Gout

The role of calcium in relation to low blood sugar and rheumatoid arthritis, as described above, also applies to many of the other conditions in the arthritis family. In osteo-arthritis, the weakened bones and muscle stiffness due, in part, to calcium imbalance, play a considerable role in the joint wear and tear. Additional factors in the low blood sugar patients are circulatory impairment, fatigue and overweight, all of which contribute to the osteo-arthritis symptoms.

Gout is closely related to arthritis and, contrary to medical thinking, it is not simply caused by an extra amount of uric acid in the blood. Dr Williams points out, 'The mere presence of high uric acid in the blood is not enough to cause gout, its salts must be precipitated in and around the joints and this does not always happen in individuals who have a high content of uric acid in the blood.'[17] This was confirmed by his finding that only one patient in ten with a high blood uric acid level showed symptoms of gout. He further showed that pantothenic acid can convert the excess uric acid into harmless, easily-excreted substances, and suggested that the individual's dietary requirements could provide the clue to this puzzling condition. Although little work has been done relating gout to low blood sugar, Joslin – the authority on diabetes – has observed that gout is very rare in diabetics.[13]

Furthermore, treatment with cortisone (a substance that we know will increase the blood sugar concentration) invariably improves the symptoms of gout.

It would be a mistake for me to suggest that arthritic conditions are entirely due to low blood sugar. Many other factors are involved, including inheritance, anaemia, stress, vitamin C levels, fats in the blood, endocrine imbalance and individual metabolic requirements. There is, however, considerable evidence available to suggest that many arthritic sufferers have associated low blood sugar, and that the treatment of the blood sugar imbalance frequently alleviates the arthritic symptoms.

8

DIABETES AND HYPOGLYCAEMIA

When discussing low blood sugar with patients in an attempt to explain its cause and treatment, I find a useful starting-point is to ask the question, 'Are you familiar with diabetes?' The usual answer is, 'Yes, although not in detail.' Even a rough understanding of diabetes aids the understanding of hypoglycaemia for, although the two conditions are opposite, the problems involved are also, in a way, complementary.

The symptoms of diabetes were noted almost 3,500 years ago, whilst hypoglycaemia was first recorded and defined a mere 50 years ago. As I have said, hypoglycaemia due to simple hyperinsulinism can be seen as an exact medical opposite to diabetes, a mirror image, as one is high blood sugar (diabetes) and the other low blood sugar (hypoglycaemia).

In order to understand how hypoglycaemia can develop into diabetes in later life, how the two conditions can exist together and why the diets prescribed for the two problems are remarkably similar, it may help to take a closer look at diabetes.

Diabetes: Its Early Study and Treatment

The excessive passing of urine, an obvious sign of diabetes, was the subject of an Egyptian papyrus written around 3,500 years ago called the Papyrus Ebeas. It gives detailed prescriptions for medicines to reduce the urine output. Close to AD 200 Aretaeus the Cappadocian produced the first precise description of diabetes. He also described tetanus, chest and heart problems and epilepsy. The word 'diabaiton' derives from the Greek word meaning 'to stand with legs apart like a ladder'. Aretaeus used this word for the symptoms of diabetes as he considered that 'the fluid uses the patient's body as a ladder to escape downwards'. The modern word 'diabetes' evolved from this original Greek word.

In the seventeenth century the word 'mellitus' (meaning honey) was added to diabetes. The Latin word for honey (mel), being the basis for mellitus, was used to describe the sweet tasting urine of the diabetic. In spite of the earlier observations, it was not until the end of the nineteenth century that some understanding of the cause of the strange symptoms of diabetes was achieved. A Russian named Oscar Minkowski showed that the removal of a dog's pancreas caused the dog to die from symptoms exactly similar to those of the diabetic sufferer.

With the field of study narrowed down to the pancreas, it was not long before workers were able to isolate the substance insulin secreted from small glands on the pancreas (later named the Islets of Langerhans) as the key to diabetes. In 1869 the glands were identified in diabetic patients. The ensuing race to discover and isolate insulin was won by a young Canadian doctor named Banting who, with his colleague Charles Best, showed that pancreatic extract (insulin) could be used to prolong the life of diabetic dogs.

The next small step involved the relatively simple process of purifying insulin for general use.

When considering diabetes one may ask, 'If the body cannot deal with sugar owing to a poor insulin response, why not simply reduce or avoid sugar and allow the pancreas to rest?' Unfortunately, we cannot avoid absorbing sugar for, although carbohydrates (starches) are completely converted to glucose, fats and proteins are also partially converted as follows.[18]

Table 4 Conversion of food groups to glucose

Food	Percentage converted
Carbohydrates	100
Fats	10
Proteins	50

It would therefore be necessary to avoid all foods if we were to prevent glucose entering the blood-stream.

When the earlier doctors treated their diabetic patients they were obliged (in the absence of insulin therapy) to adjust their patients' diet as best they could. The protein requirements are predictable and fixed and could not be safely varied as proteins are used for tissue repair, antibody production and many other vital processes. It follows that the only adjustment that could be safely achieved was to reduce carbohydrates and increase fats. The complete and safe breakdown of fats requires a minimal amount of carbohydrate and, in the type of diet prescribed to the diabetic of the pre-insulin period, there occurred an inevitable build-up of fat residues, in particular acetone and diacetic acid. This excess of acetone in the blood causes a reduction in the blood alkaline reserve and eventual coma. At the same time, acetone spills over into the urine where it can be detected. This condition is known as 'acidosis'. The acetone is also expelled via the lungs giving a characteristic smell to the breath. Before insulin was available, a diabetic patient inevitably died of acidosis, in spite of special diets and careful nursing.

Fat Absorption

An additional problem for the diabetic, and still a problem even with modern treatment, is that of fat absorption. Without insulin the liver cannot store excess sugar, which it normally does by converting the sugar to glycogen. After the liver is saturated with converted sugar (as glycogen), the excess glycogen is converted into fat and stored, usually in muscle tissue. The liver is enlarged with the deposits of stored glycogen (owing to excess consumption *or* insufficient insulin availability). Once the 'storage' areas (i.e. liver and muscle) are saturated, the excess fat overspills into the blood-stream. It is the build-up of various fats in the blood of the diabetic that leads to the two main secondary effects in mature diabetics. These are diabetic retinitis (retinopathy) and diabetic gangrene. Both these unpleasant conditions are in part due to a narrowing and thickening of small blood vessels. Not surprisingly, many diabetics are also obese owing to the store of spare fat in various tissues. High blood-pressure, strokes and heart attacks are more frequent than among non-diabetics. Other complications include athero-sclerosis, fatty livers and cataracts.

The tailoring of the insulin dosage to carbohydrate intake can, unfortunately, lead to a situation where diabetic patients need to eat more starch to balance the insulin in order to avoid 'hypo-ing' (hypoglycaemia due to excess insulin). This situation can lead to a further reduction in pancreatic efficiency, and a vicious circle is set up.

Blood Sugar Levels

The normal blood sugar fasting level is about 4-6mmol/litre of blood. However, as we are not normally fasting for periods of longer than two to three hours, it must be seen that the normal level of blood sugar during an active day would be considerably higher, i.e. 4-8mmol/litre. As the available glucose reserve in the blood is only equivalent to two teaspoonsful of sugar, it is essential for the body to be able to draw off some reserves of sugar as well as control excess sugar. The food is broken down and passed to the liver; in a similar way the insulin, when released, is also passed to the liver. This enables the small amount of insulin that remains after the excess glucose is converted to glycogen to pass throughout the body assisting the utilization of blood glucose.

We should know the events that follow the eating of carbohydrates, for then we may more easily understand high and low blood sugar conditions (see Figure 4).

If a situation arises where the blood glucose concentration exceeds 9mmol/litre, the excess spills over into the urine. This overflow level is known as the renal ('kidneys') threshold, and can be seen as a normal compensatory device to rid the blood of surplus glucose. The kidneys' 'threshold' may, however, be reduced to the point where sugar appears in the urine despite *normal* levels being present in the blood. This is known as renal diabetes and is not an expression of sugar-insulin imbalance.

At the other extreme, damaged or diseased kidneys may be unable to pass any sugar into the urine, leading to a high blood sugar level being completely masked. A true assessment of high or low blood sugar is, therefore, only obtained by measuring the blood sugar level. The most informative and valuable test is the six-hour glucose tolerance test (discussed in Chapter 11).

Adrenal Glands

There is one further piece of the jigsaw that illustrates blood sugar levels, this being the role of the adrenal glands. These glands are located near the kidneys and produce several important hormones. The centre of the gland, the medulla, secrets adrenalin (epinephrine). The outer layer, the cortex, produces cortisol (hydrocortisone), cortisone and several other less important substances. Under normal conditions, the available glucose is utilized by the body for energy and the blood glucose level drops. This lowering of blood glucose stimulates the secretions of the adrenal cortex, and the hormones released have an opposite effect to insulin. They are passed in the blood to the liver, where they facilitate the conversion of the stored glycogen into glucose. It can be seen that this balances the action of insulin and, in normal health, an optimum blood sugar level is maintained. The adrenalin secreted by the centre of the adrenal gland has a similar effect. The rate of use is, however, very different, for adrenalin can be seen as part of a 'back-up' or emergency system. It is secreted by the gland when the body requires a rapid glucose increase to provide an energy surge. The pulse then quickens and the blood-pressure rises, allowing the increased glucose to reach the muscles rapidly. In animals, this provides available energy literally for fight or flight. Unfortunately, in 'civilized' human beings, the mechanism is triggered far too frequently as a result of physical or mental stress, and the subsequent adrenal exhaustion can cause a variety of problems, in particular the lowered output of cortisone, which is related closely to the onset of joint problems, particularly rheumatoid arthritis.

To a lesser extent, the stored glycogen in the muscles is also affected by insulin and adrenal hormone levels, but the greater activity occurs in the liver.

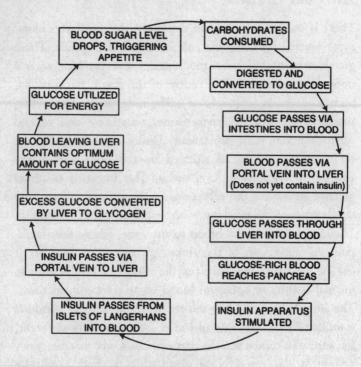

Figure 4 An outline of carbohydrate absorption

9

LOW BLOOD SUGAR OR FOOD ALLERGY?

Food allergies over the last ten years have become a much discussed and rather trendy explanation for a vast range of illnesses. In the context of this book many symptoms known to be caused by environmental or food allergies can also be caused by hypoglycaemia. The common denominators for food allergies and hypoglycaemia are as follows:

1. Diet is involved in both, whether causative or curative.

2. Both problems can show a positive GTT.[19]

3. Although the symptoms caused by allergies and low blood sugar can vary almost by the minute there is usually a pattern of symptoms associated with specific foods.

4. The symptoms of both affect the mind *and* the body, e.g. both low blood sugar and food allergy can cause fatigue but can also cause depression and anxiety.

5. Patients with either condition tend to have cravings (or even addictions) for certain food and drinks.

6. To compound the confusion, both hypoglycaemia and

food allergies can respond well to a low carbohydrate diet
with vitamin therapy.

The Cause of Allergies

The cause of food allergies is not fully understood although
Paavo Airola,[43] the American nutritionist, maintains that they
could be caused by incorrect feeding of babies under the age
of one year with cereals, meat and cow's milk for which at
that age the child lacks suitable digestive enzymes. In addition, he claims that chemical additives in foods may block or
alter biochemical pathways leading to food sensitivities. It
seems likely that allergies are an expression of our own metabolic imbalances and that allergic symptoms can be seen as
the 'side-effects' from eating common foods.

Allergy Types

There are three main types of allergy:

1. *Fixed allergy*. This involves a reaction to food every time it
   is eaten. It matters little if the food is eaten alone or with
   other food — the reaction is predictable and immediate.
   Obviously, this type of allergy is easy to identify.

2. *Build-up allergy*. Many allergic sufferers are confused to
   find that they react to a certain food one day, but not
   the next. They may have a build-up allergy and this type
   of reaction is triggered by a sensitivity to certain foods,
   but it is the *amount* of the food consumed that is critical.
   Each patient may have a different tolerance to this
   amount and when their 'trigger amount' is reached the
   symptoms develop; so they may eat bread with impunity

for 2-3 days, but bread eaten on the fourth day may cause severe symptoms. The amount needed to produce the allergy symptoms is significant, coupled with the frequency of eating. It therefore follows that if the food is avoided for a while it can again be tolerated until the critical build-up factor is reached. This type of allergy can usually be identified when the patient follows a controlled diet.

3. *Masked allergy*. This is by definition a hidden allergy, and paradoxically the allergic symptoms are controlled by repeated eating of the offending food. It is only when the food or drink is avoided that the allergic withdrawal symptoms are experienced. A person with this food addiction is usually quite unaware that this is taking place, and often the food he likes most or even craves is the substance causing the trouble. This phenomenon is not too different from the alcoholic or drug addict. Their symptoms only develop when they *stop* taking their drugs or drink. This type of allergy can usually be identified by undergoing a five-day fast.

The Diagnosis of Allergies

An interesting phenomenon of food allergies occurs when a sufferer avoids foods to which he is allergic for 4-5 days; he can become hypersensitive, suffering an acute reaction upon eating the food. This converting of a mild chronic reaction to a severe acute reaction is diagnostically useful in identifying suspect food and drinks and forms the basis for one of the most effective ways to test for food allergies. This method and others are listed below.

Diagnosis by fasting

This is perhaps one of the least stressful and certainly least expensive methods of identifying food allergies. Patients are requested to fast on bottled mineral water (glass bottles only) for at least five days to remove all food residues from the system. Alkaline salts may be recommended to clear the bowels. After this short fast, selected common foods are introduced and reactions noted. The reactions to the foods can be assessed in three ways:

(a) Symptom changes

(b) Changes in handwriting

(c) Pulse variations

In this way over a 10-12 day period patients can identify hidden allergies in most common foods by the reactions they cause, as it is usually possible to test 3-4 foods a day. This method is well described by Dr Mandell[20] and Dr Randolf[21] in their excellent books on food allergies. Both authors are prominent in the field of allergy testing and treatment in the USA.

Diagnosis by Skin Tests

This traditional method of allergy testing has been shown to be unreliable.[20] It is based on the belief that we can produce certain allergic antibodies, known as reagens, that respond to various foods tested. However, not everyone has these reagens and the characteristic 'mosquito bite' lump does not always develop. This is because many people with food sensitivities do not always react to the skin testing of foods, yet the same foods may produce symptoms when consumed. Unfortunately the converse also applies, i.e. some patients show a false positive to a skin test yet when the same substance is eaten they show no response. Clearly a confusing and unsatisfactory way of testing for food allergies.

Sublingual Testing of Allergies

This involves the testing of allergies by placing minute amounts of the suspected substance under the tongue. This is rapidly absorbed into the bloodstream and may cause a reaction. If a response occurs, it is immediate, and diagnostically available, as the symptoms produced are very similar to the actual exposure to the substance in the daily diet. Environmental allergies, dust, pollen, etc. can also be tested in this way.

Pulse Testing of Allergies

Dr Coca is a name usually associated with pulse testing and he described in the 1960s[22] his observation that the pulse rate increased when allergic foods are eaten. Although this form of testing is a little tedious it is a method that can be safely used at home. The pulse should be tested when resting and before eating the suspect food, then again at 20, 40, 60, 80 and 100 minutes after eating the food. An increase of 5 beats a minute or more is significant and the food can be double-checked if doubt exists.

Cytotoxic Testing of Allergies

This method is one of the better ways to identify food and environmental allergies. It is, however, costly (£80 plus) and very few laboratories in the UK have the necessary expertise. The patient's blood is tested by examining changes in the white cell structure and movements when the blood is exposed to selected foods, etc.[23-24] The advantages include no discomfort to patients, mild sensitivity can be detected, but perhaps the most important of all, this type of testing excludes any possibility of subjective influences, e.g. imaginary or hysterical reactions to foods. Chemicals and inhalants can also be tested in this way. The disadvantages are few, however fresh blood is required and the results depend on the skill of the laboratory staff.

Vega Testing

The Vega Test method has developed from EAV (Electro-acupuncture according to Voll). In experienced hands it is 80 to 85 per cent accurate and it offers a simple system for chemical and food sensitivity testing. The Vega Test was developed in Germany in the 1930s. This electro-acupuncture method utilises a galvanometer designed to measure the skin's electrical activity at designated points. Particular foods are placed in the 'honeycomb' in the Vega machine and if the indicator falls, this is said to demonstrate the presence of allergy to the food. Many other allergic substances can be tested in this way including inhalants, food additives and animal fur.

The method involves linking the patient to the machine via acupuncture points on the hands or feet and using electrodes in place of needles. This is a pain-free and comfortable process, and 50 to 60 suspected food substances can be tested in 60 to 90 minutes. This effective and reliable procedure does not expose patients to allergens, so there is no risk of inducing severe reactions; for this reason it is suitable for all ages, including young children.

RAST Testing (Radioallergosorbent Test)

This system involves the measuring of the levels of 1gE blood antibodies that show with specific substances such as proteins and pollens. Unfortunately, certain food compounds (such as lectins and peptides) can make the results unreliable. False food allergies can also be caused by increased sensitivity to histamine. An example of this is a magnesium deficiency affecting histamine release.

Candida Albicans – The Missing Link?

Although we may not be aware of it, we all act as hosts to a minute parasitic yeast. This fungal-like substance is related to mould and inhabits the intestine. Its full name is *Candida Albicans*, but it is usually called thrush (or Candidiasis) for this is the acute condition when candida multiplies. Our immune systems normally control Candida and a further control is the presence of competing beneficial bacteria in the human gut.

At times of stress, infection, nutritional imbalance, or the long term and regular use of the birth pill, cortisone or antibiotics, Candida proliferates and changes to a fungoid form. This changed form can damage the intestinal lining and produce a wide range of symptoms, many of which are the same as hypoglycaemia and food allergy. These include anxiety, depression, fatigue, indigestion, bowel disturbances, migraine, allergies, chronic cystitis, vaginal inflammation and infections, pruritis anni, problems of menstruation, premenstrual syndrome, skin rashes, poor memory and concentration, joint and muscle pain.

Diagnosis is not easy. Our immune system will tolerate a certain level of Candida, hence we all have a Candida population within us, therefore to identify an increase sufficient to give rise to symptoms becomes very difficult. There are, however, various clues to make one suspect a possible Candida problem. These are as follows:

1. History of cortisone or antibiotic therapy. (Both drugs tend to reduce the beneficial controlling bacteria in the intestine.)

2. An intolerance of yeast or alcohol.

3. High sugar/starch diet. (Candida feeds on sugar and sugar-rich foods.)

4. Regular use of the birth pill.

5. History of thrush or chronic cystitis.

6. Food and chemical sensitivity.

7. Symptoms of hypoglycaemia or food allergies that prove resistant to treatment.

The medical treatment for Candida is an anti-yeast drug called Nystatin. There is, however, an alternative approach which involves supporting the immune system, increasing the 'store' of beneficial intestinal bacteria, and ensuring that the diet does not provide any nutrients that will 'feed' the Candida thus reducing their growth. The following treatment procedures have been found of benefit although it may be four to six months before there is symptom relief.

1. The B vitamins biotin and folic acid help prevent conversion of the yeast Candida to the fungal form. Oleic acid (found in many oils) works the same way.

2. The immune system is strengthened by taking zinc, copper and garlic and vitamins C, A and E. All improve the mucous membranes lining the intestine. A yeast-free B complex is also of value.

3. Live *Lactobacillus Acidophilus* (in tablet or powder form) serves to replenish the depleted intestinal bacteria. This is also found in natural goat's milk yogurt.

4. Antibiotics, cortisone and similar drugs and the birth pill should be avoided if possible.

5. A hypoglycaemic-type diet is of value with certain reservations – yeast and yeast substances should be avoided. These are found in mature cheeses, vinegar, sauerkraut, alcohol, honey, oranges, pickles and yeast-based vitamins.

6. The homoeopathic remedy Candida Albicans is of value in treating Candida.

7. Caprylic acid, an extract of coconuts, is an effective anti-fungal agent. It is now available in timed-release capsules. The most commonly prescribed anti-fungal drug is Nystatin (see above). This is unfortunately yeast-based and a rebound effect can occur after the drug is discontinued, leading to a worsening of symptoms. Caprylic acid does not produce such after-effects, and it provides an excellent first stage treatment to combat Candida.

Candida is more prevalent now than 20 years ago. The incidence of food allergies, thrush, cystitis and many other symptoms is increasing. It is thought that the widespread use of antibiotics, Cortisone (and other immune-suppressive drugs) and the birth pill are contributing factors. Traces of antibiotics can be found in milk and cheese, and the food for

Candida (carbohydrate) is eaten on a vast scale in the Western nations. The differential diagnosis of hypogly-caemia, food allergies and Candida is far from easy, only careful case-history taking and detection work can identify the culprit. Unfortunately, the galaxy of seemingly uncon-nected symptoms caused by these three conditions can be very similar.

Food Allergies – Treatment

The foregoing has hopefully demonstrated to readers the link between low blood sugar and allergies. If patients are given a diagnosis of low blood sugar and the prescribed diet and treatment does not improve symptoms, the question of possible food allergies or candida infection should be investi-gated. My colleagues and I are all of the opinion, however, that many patients do not have true allergies. A simple example of this may be the migraine sufferer who predictably reacted to eating cheese with a severe migraine, yet after following a high protein diet to balance his blood sugar level and improve fat absorption he found to his delight that he could eat cheese without any symptoms.

As a general rule-of-thumb I like to approach the question of food allergies in the context of the general health. To simply identify suspect foods and exclude them from one's diet does not really answer the all-important question: 'Why is this patient sensitive to certain foods?' In my experience the required low carbohydrate diet for low blood sugar prob-lems eliminates 50 per cent to 60 per cent of so-called allergies, and the necessary back-up programme of health building that should accompany any dietary treatment frequently reduces many other food sensitivities. There are, however, cases needing detailed allergy testing and further information on this very complex subject can be obtained from the books by Drs Randolf and Mandell listed in the references [20, 21]. Your GP may be able to put you in touch with one of the specialized clinics that do allergy testing under the NHS.

Case History

Maggie, a 24-year-old airline hostess, was concerned that she suffered from multiple allergies. She experienced cravings for sugar-rich foods, with weight swings of up to 2–3kg (6–8lb) in 24 hours (especially pre-menstrually) and felt quite ill if she ate fish, eggs or chocolate. Her symptoms had persisted for 18 years and included cold hands and feet, PMS, hyperactivity, mood swings, menstrual acne and fatigue. Her appetite was unpredictable but usually poor and she always experienced relief when eating sugar. Without sugar for more than three or four hours, she trembled and felt very weak. She was 16kg (2½ stones) overweight.

Her first test was a comprehensive Vega check, which showed no response. A hair mineral analysis indicated low levels of chromium, calcium, iron, magnesium, manganese, potassium selenium and zinc. A six-hour glucose tolerance test confirmed a severe reactive curve with a 4.5mmol/litre fasting figure and a fall to 1.6mmol/litre during the test.

The family history was significant. Her father and brother suffered from migraine, her sister was a hay-fever sufferer and her other sister experienced similar symptoms to Maggie.

Maggie's diet was a little unusual consisting of one meal daily (usually pasta) and many snacks of crisps, biscuits, sweets and fruit; with approximately 15 to 20 cups of sweet coffee over 24 hours.

The hypoglycaemic diet was prescribed with B-complex and adrenal and thyroid glandular support to step-up metabolic *activity. She was also advised to take extra vitamin B$_6$ and zinc.*

In spite of her worst fears, she lost 4½ kg (10lb) in the first six weeks and has continued to lose at the rate of ½–1 kg (1½–2lb) weekly. After nine months she is now symptom-free and is able to enjoy food she has not eaten for many years. Unfortunately, she still has the occasional sugar craving before periods, but is able to resist temptations.

10

LOW BLOOD SUGAR: THE 20th CENTURY EPIDEMIC

'Epidemic' is defined in the *Oxford Dictionary* as 'prevalent among community at special time'. The symptoms and illness caused by low blood sugar are certainly prevalent among the community, the special time being the twentieth century. Considerable debate surrounds the question of whether hypoglycaemia is a common condition expressed in a multiple of disorders, or a very rare condition that is falsely blamed for the disorders. The answer to this question surely lies in the frequency of diagnosis of hypoglycaemia. Doctors who regularly use glucose tolerance tests as a diagnostic tool have offered figures ranging from 10-50 per cent of the population for the incidence of hypoglycaemia. Data from a 1966-7 survey carried out by the US Department of Health, Education and Welfare showed that some 66,000 persons from a total of 134,000 were hypoglycaemic.[25] When Dr C. R. Harper tested 175 United Airlines pilots, 44 showed evidence of hypoglycaemia.[26] Dr Atkins, the American authority on nutrition and disease, who has tested many thousands of patients with the six-hour glucose tolerance test, has found that one in ten patients has been diagnosed as hypoglycaemic.[27] More will be said about the glucose tolerance test and the diagnosis of hypoglycaemia in later chapters. Sufficiently to say, however, that this condition is certainly not rare.

This chapter deals with the many less obvious conditions that can be caused by hypoglycaemia. Most of them are on the increase in 'civilized' countries.

Sugar Consumption

The great diseases of the previous centuries, e.g. tuberculosis, smallpox, cholera, syphilis, diphtheria and typhoid have been virtually eliminated, but this century has seen an increase in the degenerative and mental disorders. Diabetes, asthma, rheumatoid arthritis, heart conditions, cancer, obesity and mental illnesses are all increasing and can be seen as the characteristic diseases of this century. It is significant that the increased incidence of these conditions correlates with the increased sugar consumption in this century.

Although it should be stated that other factors may also cause these disorders, there is much evidence to show that declining health affects a country or community when sugar consumption increases. Dr T. L. Cleave has described conditions caused by taking excess sugar as the 'saccharine disease'.[28] He has shown that the introduction of sugar to primitive societies in various parts of the world has resulted in a rapid increase in diabetes (which so often follows hypoglycaemia), stomach ulcers and coronary heart disease. He has observed that the increased consumption of sugar in Western nations causes a corresponding increase in mortality from diabetes. (In the Metropolitan Life Insurance Company's causes of death statistics, diabetes in 1900 was twenty-seventh on the list. By 1950 it was the third most common cause of death.) Dr Cleave states that, '. . . the key to the causation of coronary thrombosis lies in the causation of diabetes'.

The Heart and Hypoglycaemia

Coronary heart disease is now the number one killer. How can it be that a condition which a mere century ago was attributed to old age and therefore rarely mentioned in medical text books is now responsible for the death of tens of thousands of apparently healthy men and women, many of whom were in their late twenties and thirties? The answer lies in the massive increase in the consumption of sugar and the imbalance in sugar and fat metabolism that results from this consumption. A lot of research has been carried out to show that hypoglycaemia and a high sugar diet contribute to various heart disorders. In 1933 Dr Paton wrote in *The Lancet* that the rise in sugar consumption may be the cause of heart disease and heart attacks. He pointed out that the 'clinically associated' conditions of obesity, arterio-sclerosis and diabetes are also on the increase. Dr R. A. Ahrens of the University of Maryland showed conclusively in a number of animal studies that increased sugar consumption shortened the average life-span.[29] He added weight to the cholesterol myth by concluding that the huge worldwide increase in heart disease increases in rough proportion to the increase in sugar consumption, and not fat consumption.

The heart specialists, White and Stare, wrote in 1954, 'No disease has come so quickly from obscurity to the place coronary heart disease now occupies.' (i.e. Heart disease is the primary cause of death in the USA.) Many workers have shown the correlation between hypoglycaemia and the incidence of heart disease, including Dr B. Sandler. His paper in the *Homeostasis* (Autumn, 1974)[30] showed that angina and coronary heart disease are frequently caused by a sharp fall in the blood sugar level.

CHOLESTEROL

Surely a word to strike terror in most people. For years it has been blamed as the single main cause of heart disease. As a result, patients have been encouraged to reduce the fat in their diet to dangerously low levels, and to avoid valuable protein foods. Yet to date, no evidence is available to show that eating cholesterol actually affects our blood cholesterol levels. Indeed, many patients with an inherited high cholesterol level have perfectly sound hearts, and many coronary victims have normal cholesterol levels.

It has long been assumed that most overweight people have an imbalance in their carbohydrate metabolism. Insulin is sometimes called the fattening hormone simply because it promotes the storage of starch and fat. (The stored starch is known as glycogen and the stored fat is termed triglycerides.) Insulin also converts fatty acids back to stored fat. Not surprisingly, those of us with hypoglycaemia and hyperinsulinism tend to be overweight. So the patient with low blood sugar craves sugar, the high sugar diet produces insulin which causes fat to be stored and eventually spill over into the blood. Finally the excessive insulin creates low blood sugar and so the craving for sugar continues.

TRIGLYCERIDES

In 1958 Kinsall showed that the circulating saturated fats (triglycerides) were a main factor in clotting in heart attacks and not, as was suspected, the level of cholesterol. Of 100 patients who suffered heart attacks as a result of clots, only 18 per cent had blood cholesterol levels in excess of 6.8mmol/litre (normal range 3.6-6.8mmol/litre), while almost 90 per cent had an abnormally high level of trigly-cerides. It is interesting to learn that if a person with high blood fat level is under stress, the storage fat is released into the blood by the action of the adrenal hormones, and the blood fat levels can increase dramatically.

KETOSIS

In a typical diet, half our energy is supplied from starch or sugar, the remaining half is provided by protein and fat. If we avoid carbohydrate completely and consume fat and protein only, our body uses stored carbohydrate (glycogen) as food. This supply is, however, used up within two to three days. After this time, the body fat is utilized and the main storage fat (triglyceride) is broken down into free fatty acids and 'ketones'. When fat is broken down in this way, so that the two fuels (fatty acids and ketones) are present in the blood, the process is known as *ketosis*. Many weight reducing diets are aimed at producing mild ketosis to burn off excessive fat. (Diabetics, however, can develop a more serious form of ketosis which can cause dangerous weight loss.) This contro-versial diet is called the ketogenic diet and is prescribed for a range of problems including hypoglycaemia, epilepsy and schizophrenia.

I have found in practice that a balanced wholefood diet, high in fresh fruit and vegetables and avoiding starch, is quite effective for reducing high levels of triglycerides and choles-terol in the blood. This is without insisting that patients avoid the cholesterol-rich foods (eggs, cheese, etc.) which are important sources of protein, vitamins, minerals and fats. Research has shown that to avoid cholesterol completely can be hazardous as it is an essential constituent of many hormones and assists the absorption of food. A low choles-terol diet can also have the unfortunate effect of stimulating the body to produce more cholesterol as only 20 per cent of our total cholesterol is provided by the food we eat. Unsaturated vegetable fats and phospholipids (lecithin) are of value in aiding utilization and transport of fat by clearing the fat deposited in the cells through the body. As we will see later when discussing treatment, this diet is virtually the same as the hypoglycaemic diet, and for this reason is of double value for the heart sufferer.

Mental Health[69]

This covers a vast array of topics ranging from suicide and crime to schizophrenia, anxiety and addictions. The mechanism whereby an inadequate supply of glucose to the brain cells can lead to personality disorders has been covered in previous chapters. It may, however, be of interest to delve a little deeper to show how poor nutrition and, in particular, low blood sugar, can affect the mind.

There is a tendency to attribute the great increase in mental illness over the last 50 years to the stressful effects of modern society. Sociologists and psychiatrists point to the damaging effects of television whereby the harrowing and distressing news from all over the world is introduced into our own homes. The economic pressures and competitiveness of society are blamed for the high incidence of anxiety neurosis, depression and nervous breakdowns. The consumption of tranquillizers and antidepressants is increasing year by year, and alcoholism and drug addiction is growing at an alarming rate. Anti-social behaviour and crimes of all types are also increasing. Can we really lay the blame for all this upon the pace of modern society? Surely there have been times in man's history when there was an equivalent or even greater degree of stress upon the individual? One has only to read Dickens, Zola or Tolstoy to appreciate the great despair and unhappiness that the majority of people experienced in previous centuries.

Do other, less advanced, cultures suffer the same mental problems as our own, and have the effects of stress in relation to nutrition ever been investigated in laboratory trials? Although there are no cut-and-dried answers to these questions, it may help to look a little closer at the history of stress in the hope that another explanation for the present epidemic of nervous ailments can be found.

Dr R. Williams, world famous chemist and nutritionist, wrote some years ago, 'The brain cells ultimately get from the blood only those nutrient elements that are furnished in the food we eat.'[17] Perhaps, for many of us, this is an obvious statement, yet it is the work of Roger Williams, Linus Pauling and other nutritionists and researchers who have paved the way for a more empirical explanation for mental disease, based not on altered personality and Freudian complexes, but on the bio-chemical requirements and nutritional imbalances within the brain and nervous system.

For many years it was assumed that vitamins, minerals and trace elements were needed by the body only in minute quantities, and that these quantities were adequately supplied by the normal Western diet. Roger Williams has, however, shown that individual requirements for certain substances vary enormously, and there are those who need ten to twenty times the average requirement of certain substances, just to maintain normal health. Dr Williams' book *Biochemical Individuality*[31] has caused a rethinking by the more enlightened health workers on the whole question of vitamin deficiency and the normal daily requirements of many substances. The book explains that many people suffer from mild vitamin deficiencies that give rise to personality disorders. This phenomenon is termed 'sub-clinical' as the more gross symptoms of pellagra, scurvy, rickets, etc. are not present. Dr Williams logically assumed that, between the so-called healthy individuals and those suffering from gross deficiency states, are many layers of mild deficiencies, often due not to deficient diets but to some individuals requiring huge amounts of vitamins not available in the typical diet. If we look at the symptoms of some of the vitamin deficient states (particularly Vitamin B), we can see that the *earliest* symptoms of deficiency usually involve the mind before physical symptoms show.

Vitamin B_1/Thiamine. The earliest deficiency symptoms include neurasthenia, depression, poor memory, fatigue, poor concentration, vague stomach and heart symptoms.

Vitamin B_3/Niacin, Nicotinic Acid, Nicotinamide. Earliest deficiency symptoms include neurasthenia, confusion, anxiety, fear, depression accompanied by skin, mouth and other ailments.

Vitamin C. Earliest symptoms of deficiency including bruising, poor healing, irritability, anxiety and depression.

Biotin. Earliest symptoms include fatigue, insomnia and anorexia.

Pantothenic Acid. Earliest deficiency symptoms include fatigue, apathy, depression, muscular weakness.

A great deal of research on animals and humans has confirmed that inadequate nutrition can have an affect upon the mind. Fortunately, in the early stages at least, these effects are reversible. In addition to depression and anxiety, actual personality changes have been recorded when subjects

have agreed to follow vitamin-deficient diets, the old personality reappearing as the diet is normalized. Table 5 on page
88 gives a complete list of nutrients particularly relevant to
mental health, and shows the variety of emotional conditions
caused by a diet deficient in these nutrients.

Other factors influencing the effects of nutrition on
the brain environment include drug side-effects, tobacco,
alcohol, food additives, etc. When discussing nutrition to
the brain, it should be remembered that the availability of
adequate glucose to nerve tissue is essential for the efficient
transport, absorption and utilization of many essential nutrients. Lewis showed in 1974[32] with animal tests that hypoglycaemia produced lethargy and weariness due to lowered
absorption of essential brain nutrients. In the same journal,
Lewis showed that hypoglycaemia can cause a decrease in the
tissue concentration of most citric acid cycle (Krebs Cycle)
components.[33] Vitamin B_1, pantothenic acid, Vitamin B_2 and
B_3, are all closely involved with this cycle which is the 'major
route of carbohydrate metabolism in the body[34] and is fundamental to our energy needs'. It has also been shown that
hypoglycaemia causes a decreased oxygen availability to brain
tissue with resulting biochemical inefficiency.

Much work is still to be done on the connection between
nutrition and the mind, but it is becoming clear that an
optimum supply of blood sugar is vital for normal mental
health.

CASE HISTORY

*Mike was a self-employed company director aged 48. For no
apparent reason he developed symptoms of depression, breathlessness, anxiety and fatigue for which his GP had prescribed Ativan
over the previous three years, putting his symptoms down to work
pressures. This drug-reliance concerned Mike who claimed that he*

had 'no real worries'. Significantly, he always felt worse in the morning, becoming particularly anxious, even dizzy, when driving the five miles to work.

His diet was as follows:

Breakfast	Toast and marmalade, 2 cups of tea (2 spoons of sugar in each)
11 a.m.	Cup of tea, crisps or cheese roll
Lunch	Chips, roll, tea
3 p.m.	Tea and biscuits
Dinner	Usual English meal followed by tea
Supper	(About 10–11p.m.) Coffee and biscuits
Alcohol	Nil
Smoking	20 cigarettes daily
Chocolate	Daily

A hair mineral analysis showed low levels of chromium, magnesium, manganese, zinc and potassium. The six-hour glucose tolerance test produced a fasting level of 4.8mmol/litre with a fall to 2.3mmol/litre. A low-sugar, low-starch diet was advised and Mike was requested to reduce his cigarettes. A glandular adrenal support was prescribed with a multi-mineral and vitamin B-complex. Vitamin C was also advised to offset the effects of smoking.

Over a period of three to four months the diet and other measures stabilized the blood sugar slump in the mornings, and Mike is now off the Ativan and feeling more relaxed and vital.

Cancer

One person in every four in Europe and America will, at some time in his or her life, develop cancer. Although there are many different types of cancer, depending on location and tissue affected, there is growing evidence available to show a positive link between blood sugar levels and certain types of cancer.

The statistical evaluation of what, in America, is called DDDs (diabetes detection drives), when coupled with the patient's history of tumours, provided significant information which can be summarized as follows:

1. The risk of cancer increases as we get older.

2. People below 29 years reported no history of cancer.

3. Those in the 30-50 years age bracket with hypoglycaemia reported most cancer.

4. In the oldest age group, 50 and over, the incidence of cancer closely paralleled the incidence of diabetes.

5. In all ages, overweight directly related to cancer incidence.

These susceptibility tests were carried out at the University of Alabama Medical Center by Dr Cheraskin and colleagues.[35] They concluded that the causes leading to hypoglycaemia and later, diabetes, were all contributive causes of cancer. It therefore follows that early detection and treatment of hypoglycaemia is one way to contribute to cancer prevention.

Alcoholism

It may seem out of place to include a section on alcoholism on a book on low blood sugar. There is, however, a strong connection between the two, and a reciprocal relationship exists between alcohol and blood sugar. Alcoholism can

Table 5 Effects of nutritional deficiencies on the mind

Nutrient	Effects
Vitamin B$_3$ (niacin, nicotinic acid, nicotinamide) deficiency	Insomnia, nervousness, irritability, confusion, apprehensiveness, depression, hallucination.
Vitamin B$_1$ (thiamine) deficiency	Loss of appetite, depression, irritability, confusion, memory loss, inability to concentrate, sensitivity to noise.
Vitamin B$_2$ (riboflavin) deficiency	Depression.
Pantothenic acid deficiency	Depression, unable to tolerate stress.
Vitamin B$_6$ (pyridoxine) deficiency	Abnormal responses in psychotic children.
Vitamin B$_{12}$ deficiency	Difficulty in concentration and remembering, stuporous depression, severe agitation, hallucinations, manic or paranoid behaviour.
Biotin deficiency	Depression, lassitude, panic, hallucinations.
Vitamin C administration	Improvement on schizophrenia.
Niacin supplement	Improvement in schizophrenia.
Iodine deficiency	Cretinism.
Potassium deficiency	Nervousness, irritability, mental disorientation.
Magnesium deficiency	Paranoid psychosis.
Threonine deficiency	Irritability, hard to get along with.
Lysine deficiency	Inability to concentrate.
Glutamic acid administration	Improvement in intelligence and general brain functioning in mental retardation.
Folic acid supplement	Improvement in psychosis.
Lactate excess in blood	Anxiety, neurosis, fatigue, insomnia, tension.
Calcium deficiency	Anxiety, neurosis, fatigue, insomnia, tension.

cause hypoglycaemia, and many experts accept that there is a condition known as alcohol-induced hypoglycaemia. Dr Tintera, an expert on alcoholism and blood sugar, has stated that 'Low blood sugar is central to the alcoholic problem.'

As described in Chapter 5, the symptoms of a hangover are due to hypoglycaemia. Unfortunately, these symptoms are, for the alcoholic, chronic and recurring. The effect of alcohol is to lower the output of glucose by the liver, so triggering off a worsening existing hypoglycaemia. Conversely, the hypoglycaemic sufferer drinks because alcohol has the same effect as sugar.

In an interesting experiment laboratory rats were divided into two groups. One group was provided with a high carbohydrate 'junk' diet, the other with a biologically ideal diet. Both groups were given a choice of water or alcohol to the drink. The first group with the high sugar diet turned to alcohol for drink, while their better-fed neighbours drank only water. These animals were not under stress, resentful, depressed, unhappy or frustrated. They just turned willingly to alcohol when their diet was inadequate. Furthermore, they became reformed alcoholics when their diets were improved and their carbohydrate level reduced.

In alcoholism a vicious circle develops with the alcohol providing a temporary uplift only to be followed by hypoglycaemia, until eventually only regular drinking achieves any comfort or relief. Alcoholics who succeed in drying out usually substitute sweets. They are still in a vicious circle, but perhaps a more socially acceptable one. Research has shown that the majority of alcoholics had a high sugar intake before the heavy drinking started, many craving sugar and sweet food as children. The withdrawal symptoms of dry mouth, sweating and tremors experienced by the reformed alcoholics are, in part, due to an inability to correct their low blood sugar condition. This is aggravated by the habit of ex-alcoholics to eat sugar and chocolate when they experience these 'jitters'. Many reformed alcoholics who are, it is claimed, psychologically cured, have relapses owing to a continuing imbalance in their blood sugar. Simply to shift from alcohol to sugar is not the complete answer. The real answer once more lies in solving – through diet and other rational treatment – the underlying hypoglycaemia.

Drug Addiction

It is not a great step from alcoholism to drug addiction. Clinical studies by Dr Tintera have shown that alcoholics often become barbiturate addicts, and many heroin addicts have a positive glucose tolerance test result confirming hypoglycaemia. As with the alcoholic, the drug addict cannot usually afford good nutrition owing, in part, to the high cost of drugs, but also his abnormal craving for drugs replaces nutrition.

Many readers will be surprised to learn that there is a drug consumed on a daily basis by most of us which can cause great physical and emotional damage. That drug is caffeine.

CAFFEINISM

Also called 'coffee nerves', this condition has long been incorrectly thought of as psychological. Work by Dr J. Greder,[36] Director of the Walker Reed US Army Medical Centre, has shown that around 250mg of caffeine are sufficient to cause symptoms of caffeinism. These include shaking, headaches, anxiety, restlessness and lethargy. Table 6 shows the caffeine content of typical food, drinks and drugs. It will be seen that to consume 250mg would not be difficult or unusual. The figures are approximate.

Table 6 Caffeine content of typical foods[17]

Food	Caffeine Content
Chocolate bar	160mg per 8 oz (225g)
Aspirin-based tablets	15-30mg each
Coffee	100-150mg per cupful
Tea	60-75 mg per cupful
Cola drinks	40-60mg per cupful

I have frequently encountered patients whose gross daily intake of caffeine is in excess of 1500mg.

Caffeine has an effect similar to sugar, although its action is not so immediate. It stimulates the adrenal glands to increase the blood sugar level, with a subsequent release of insulin to balance the sugar increase. For this reason, caffeine can act as a temporary stimulant to keep one awake. As with many other drugs, unpleasant withdrawal symptoms are experienced if the heavy coffee drinker attempts to stop the habit. Where there is a low tolerance of caffeine, anxiety and other emotional symptoms may be felt when consuming only two to three cups of coffee daily.

The addictive properties of caffeine in coffee have been investigated by many authorities. It has been demonstrated that coffee addicts show the recognizable signs of addiction. These are:

1. Able to tolerate coffee.

2. Unpleasant withdrawal symptoms when discontinuing.

3. A craving for coffee if deprived.

Caffeine produces a 'lift'. It creates a need in a similar way to alcohol, nicotine and a whole range of habit-forming substances. In the context of hypoglycaemia it constitutes a part of a vicious circle and, for this reason, caffeine, in the form of strong tea, coffee, chocolate or cola drinks, is totally banned from hypoglycaemia diets. I try to encourage patients to grow to like decaffeinated coffee and mild herbal teas.

TOBACCO

By now you will be accusing me of being a killjoy. What is there left? Is nothing sacred? Nicotine creates a shockwave in the blood sugar levels. Rises of 36-75 per cent in the blood glucose level have been shown in some studies. This is due to stimulation of the adrenal glands by the nicotine, rapidly followed by a drop in the glucose level. This see-saw effect explains the chain smoker's dilemma, for after each cigarette he craves another pick-up. Unfortunately, smoking creates a desire for caffeine, sweet foods and alcohol (smokers drink more often than non-smokers, indeed, the incidence of heavy drinking in smokers and non-smokers is in the proportion of two to one). The withdrawal symptoms are once more very similar to hypoglycaemic symptoms, i.e., headaches, drowsiness, trembling, anxiety and palpitations. Not surprisingly, smoking is a handicap in the treatment of hypoglycaemia, for often patients follow the correct diet but their symptoms do not change. There are two reasons for this:

1. Adrenal stimulation from nicotine constantly triggers the release of glucose into the blood.

2. Smoking is known to cause vitamin C loss. The rate of loss has been set at around 25mg per cigarette.[27] As this vitamin is connected with sugar metabolism controls, its value for the hypoglycaemic is indisputable.

There are obviously more serious health risks for the alcoholic, drug addict and heavy smoker than reactive hypoglycaemia. Owing to the reciprocal relationship of cause and effect with all these substances and hypoglycaemia, it can do nothing but good for the health of the 'user' to look to his or her nutrition to rebalance glucose levels and, with luck, 'kick the habit'.

Epilepsy

One of the many conditions that hypoglycaemia can mimic is epilepsy, also known as 'grand mal' or 'petit mal', depending on its severity. There are many types of epilepsy classified according to cause and symptoms. In the context of epilepsy due to hypoglycaemia I am referring chiefly to petit mal, the symptoms of which range from slight dizzy spells lasting several seconds to prolonged blackouts.

As long ago as the 1920s it was known that Islet tumours (tumours of the Islets of Langerhans – glands of the pancreas) caused convulsions and epileptic-type symptoms owing to insulin oversecretion. Removal of the tumours in most cases cured the patient of these symptoms. In 1947 Fabrykant noted that the EEG patterns of epileptics were remarkably similar to those of the hypoglycaemic patients. For many years it has been known that epileptics tested with a six-hour glucose tolerance test often show a positive low blood sugar result.

Other clues are available to show the relationship between hypoglycaemia and epilepsy:

1. Pregnant epileptics often have fewer epileptic episodes or attacks, possibly owing to the higher blood sugar during pregnancy.

2. Many young epileptics have a craving for sweet foods and drinks, and the timing of epileptic attacks often coincides with the time when the blood sugar would be low, e.g. on rising and when meals are missed.

3. Stress, whether mental or physical (e.g. through taking coffee and sugar) have been known to trigger off an epileptic attack. As we know, stress also reduces the blood sugar level.

4. The diet usually prescribed for hypoglycaemics reduces epileptic symptoms.

Other factors are known to contribute to epileptic attacks, not least the role of calcium, magnesium and vitamin B_6 (pyridoxine). There seems little doubt, however, that when the complex process whereby glucose and its derivatives are made available to brain cells is thrown off balance by hypoglycaemia, epilepsy may be one of the results.

Stomach Ulcers

Reactive hypoglycaemia is thought to be partly caused by what is termed 'uncomplicated hyperinsulinism'. This is an excess of insulin in the blood due to an overactivity of the insulin apparatus. Although many glandular influences are involved, the end result is too much insulin and not enough sugar.

Studies have shown that hypoglycaemia causes a stimulus to the vagus nerve leading to increased secretion of gastric acids.[38] It is of interest to learn that the method of testing this reaction is to inject patients (animal and human) with intravenous insulin. The German workers Feurle, Arnold, Eydt et al wrote in 1973 that '. . . this rise in gastrin occurred fifteen minutes after the lowered blood sugar level had been reached and was accompanied by an abrupt rise in hydrochloric acid concentration'.[39]

If we refer to a friend or colleague as a 'real ulcer case' we are referring to a certain type of stressful personality. It is generally accepted that severe mental and nervous stress can contribute to stomach ulcers. Dr Hans Seyle states examples of ulcers developing in a matter of days during the war before combat or after air raids.[16] The stomach wall becomes ulcerated owing to an inappropriate increase in stomach acid that is released either when no food is present in the stomach or is simply released in excessive quantities. In either case the stomach can literally digest itself.

The ulcer is perhaps the most common and obvious example of how the mind can affect the body. Unfortunately, the ulcer victim also suffers owing to the faulty breakdown in the absorption of food components, in particular protein, certain vitamins, calcium, etc. This tends to perpetuate his problems and his anxiety.

As with diabetics and asthma, the incidence of diabetic patients also having ulcers is very low, and diabetics with ulcers who have been tested with a glucose tolerance test have been found to have dysinsulinism (fluctuating between high and low blood sugar). Abrahamson[18] tested 16 ulcer patients with a six-hour glucose tolerance test. All the patients had typical ulcer symptoms, i.e. heartburn and pain, etc. and the diagnosis of ulcers had been previously confirmed by X-ray findings. All the 16 showed conclusive signs of hypoglycaemia.

Because there are so many interrelated factors when considering the cause of ulcers, it is not possible to say that hypoglycaemia is the sole cause. Many ulcer patients do not exhibit the typical hypoglycaemic symptoms. It seems likely, however, that by the same token stress is not the sole cause and is invariably accompanied by dietary considerations. The intake of protein, coffee, nicotine, vitamins and many drugs all affect the stomach acid. If stress alone is the cause of ulcers, why was the incidence of stomach ulcers higher in American training camps in World War Two than in the actual fighting units in combat conditions? Abrahamson believes this paradox is due to the greater consumption of caffeine contained in soft drinks and coffee in the training camps. The high-starch Western diet has resulted in a huge increase in the incidence of stomach ulcers. Dr Cleave states in his book *The Peptic Ulcer*[40] that the incidence of peptic ulcers parallels the intake of refined starches. He believes that over several million years of evolution man has learned how to deal with stress and, for this reason, it is not a causative factor in ulcer production.

Perhaps the answer lies somewhere between the nutrition and the stress schools of thought. Once more in the hypoglycaemia story we are presented with a vicious circle — incorrect diet and stress leading to hypoglycaemia which leads to further stress and dietary imbalance owing to the ulcer symptoms. The circle is complete.

The treatment of the ulcer patient is very similar to the many other conditions caused by hypoglycaemia, and the stressful symptoms that contribute to the problem are often also relieved.

CASE HISTORY

Roger was a taxi driver aged 56. For 25 years he had suffered stomach pain, wind and bloating after meals. This was diagnosed as acid stomach or nervous stomach, coupled with the reassurance that he did not have an ulcer. Symptoms usually developed 1½ to 2 hours after eating and were worse under stress or when fatigued.

The treatment had consisted of anti-acids with very little advice on what to eat. The nature of his work encouraged 'snack' eating with a high starch/sugar diet and 12 to 15 cups of coffee daily. On night shift he usually ate chips or chocolate bars. Not surprisingly, he was 3 stones overweight.

A six-hour glucose tolerance test was requested and showed a fasting level of 4.5mmol/litre with a fall during the test to 2.6mmol/litre. Roger was prescribed the hypoglycaemic diet but with an emphasis towards the 'food-combining' or Hay Diet. This involved separating carbohydrates from proteins to facilitate a more efficient digestion. In addition, he was prescribed a two-phase digestive enzyme to be taken in tablet form before each meal. This formula contained betaine, glutamic acid, pepsin, papain, pancreatin, pancrelipase, amylase, bromelain, ox bile and raw parotid.

Although Roger found it difficult to relax during work, the relief obtained from the above programme improved his stomach symptoms and he generally had more energy. He also lost 12½kg (2 stones) in weight.

Obesity

Hypoglycaemia has been called the 'hunger disease'. The fluctuations in blood sugar levels cause frequent hunger pangs that are relieved only by constantly overeating. The inevitable consequence of this is overweight, for unless the consumption of carbohydrates is balanced by a very high energy output (as in the case of the athlete or the labourer), the excess carbohydrate is converted to glycogen and stored in the liver and muscles. We know that hypoglycaemia, whether expressed as alcoholism, stomach ulcers or anxiety neurosis, is invariably temporarily relieved by taking more sugar. For this reason there is a close relationship between

overweight and hypoglycaemia. It has been estimated that 20
per cent of the population are overweight. The obese person
who 'must' have a chocolate, the alcoholic who 'must' have
one more drink, are probably suffering from the same withdrawal symptoms brought about by low blood sugar.

Insulin is the only hormone in the body that promotes
the storage of fuel. For this reason it is often termed the
'fattening hormone'. It converts and stores carbohydrate to
glycogen and fat to triglyceride. So hypoglycaemia promotes
fat and overweight in two ways:

1. The excessive insulin invariably found in hypoglycaemia
   causes the body to deposit fat in the tissues.

2. Hypoglycaemia increases hunger and sugar craving.

Except for thyroid imbalance and certain rare metabolic
defects, overweight is caused by overeating. The problem in
the overweight person is not one of what to eat and what
diet to follow; the calorie-controlled or carbohydrate unit-
controlled diets are readily available. The problem lies in
self-control in overcoming the almost overpowering craving
to eat. Unfortunately for the hypoglycaemic, the urge to eat
high sugar foods causes more weight increase. It is essential,
however, that the overweight patient considers every aspect
of weight control: simply to follow a 500-600 calorie diet
could be disastrous. Thyroid output may need to be checked
and the effects of fluid retention due to a variety of causes
should not be overlooked.

Hypoglycaemia leads to stress with subsequent potassium
loss and sodium retention. This causes a waterlogging of
tissues known as oedema. For many reasons, simply to
reduce food intake is not always the answer. What is often

required is an interim period to resolve the blood sugar imbalance, thyroid imbalance or fluid imbalance before dieting commences. If your weight is not reduced by a 1000-calories-a-day diet then advice should be sought on the many possible reasons for overweight.

It is generally accepted that overweight is an adverse complication in many conditions relating to hypoglycaemia, including osteo-arthritis, heart disease and diabetes.

CASE HISTORY

Many patients with low blood sugar are overweight. Their fatigue slows their metabolism and their appetite encourages over-eating, particularly of high-calorie starches and sugars.

Irene was a 52-year-old dressmaker. Although only 1.57m (5'2") tall she weighed 105kg (16½ stones). She was always tired, suffered frequent headaches and had very cold hands and feet. A hair mineral analysis showed low levels of chromium, calcium, magnesium, manganese, potassium and zinc. A six-hour glucose tolerance test showed a 'flat fatigue curve' with a fasting level of 2.7mmol/litre, falling to a low point of 1.3mmol/litre. Not surprisingly Irene craved sugar, her diet was almost exclusively starch and she consumed 36 to 40 teaspoons of sugar daily in teas and coffees, and 113–170 gms (4-6oz) of chocolate daily. She had battled with her weight for many years, and although she lost some weight with 800 to 1000 calorie diets, the subsequent weight gain was always faster than the weight loss.

She was prescribed the usual hypoglycaemic diet. This caused initial horror because of the high protein/fat content. However, she began to feel better and lost 6lb after 2 weeks. Her 'basal' temperature (underarm, morning temperatures) averaged 96.4°F over four days. She was therefore prescribed a hormone-free thyroid support, coupled with a multi-vitamin and multi-mineral formula. Irene's temperature normalized at 98°F after three

*months and her weight after six months was 73kg (11½ stones).
Her sugar craving was considerably reduced and her headaches
had cleared. She also had a lot more energy, and for the first time
for many years no longer had cold hands and feet.*

Neuralgia

As you may recall from previous discussion, hypoglycaemia
can cause swelling and pressure around blood vessels due
to vasodilation. This compensatory mechanism can lead to
headaches, particularly migraine. I have observed, however,
that another equally stubborn condition can be caused or
aggravated by hypoglycaemia, that is trigeminal neuralgia –
or tic douloureux. The trigeminal nerve is one of a group of
twelve nerves known as the cranial nerves. It branches into
three nerves, which in turn pass to the forehead and the eye
region, the cheek and the jaw. The neuralgia can involve
any combination of these three nerves and can be, at times,
very severe and resistant to treatment. Trigeminal sufferers
frequently experience an aggravation of their symptoms
shortly after eating sweet foods, in a similar way to the
migraine sufferers. I have therefore found that diet along the
lines of the hypoglycaemia diet has often proved of benefit.

Quite apart from the possible local pressure due to vasodilation (as in migraine) hypoglycaemia can cause calcium
reduction in the blood, creating a general irritability of the
nervous system (see Chapter 7). This would no doubt
contribute to neuralgia symptoms anywhere in the body.

Multiple Sclerosis

A little understood aspect of the influence of blood sugar
changes on muscle and nerve tissue is the role of hypo-

glycaemia in multiple sclerosis. Muscular weakness, poor co-ordination, subjective coldness and paraesthesia (pins and needles) with general lethargy, are symptoms common to hypoglycaemia and multiple sclerosis. Some researchers have attempted to show a link between multiple sclerosis and gluten intolerance, this hypothesis being supported by the symptom-improvement achieved by multiple sclerosis patients when following a prescribed gluten-free diet (essentially avoidance of wheat products). It would, however, seem more than likely that this type of diet also produces a temporary rebalancing of a low blood sugar situation and, if this is the case, it is not the gluten alone that contributes to the symptoms but all forms of cereal and carbohydrate. Many multiple sclerosis sufferers are sensitive to cereals and sugar, and obtain a measure of symptom-relief on the standard hypoglycaemic diet. I routinely recommend that multiple sclerosis patients undergo a six-hour glucose tolerance test, and the majority do in fact show clear signs of low blood sugar.

CASE HISTORY

Janet was a 30-year-old housewife with a diagnosis of multiple sclerosis. The symptoms of blurred vision, lethargy, muscle weakness and paraesthesia in one arm (pins and needles) had developed six years previously. Significantly, she also had a history of migraine. Her mother was a migraine sufferer and her brother has asthma.

Her six-hour glucose tolerance test showed a flat curve associated with poor absorption, the fasting level being 3.7mmol/litre with a low point of 2.2mmol/litre. The hair mineral analysis showed very low levels of magnesium and zinc. With moderately low levels of chromium and potassium. A Vega check was negative. Janet's diet was average, but she drank 10 to 12 sweet coffees and smoked 20 cigarettes daily.

She was placed on the hypoglycaemic diet and advised to stop _smoking and avoid coffee. In addition, she was prescribed a multi-mineral and a vitamin B-complex. She was also given 2½mg injection of vitamin B_{12} weekly and 1g of evening primrose oil in capsule form daily. Janet was also given a course of osteopathic treatment to mobilize her neck and spine, and acupuncture to reduce paraesthesia._

She began to feel better after two months and became virtually symptom-free after four months. Although spontaneous remissions are not unusual in multiple-sclerosis, Janet's case demonstrated the value of a 'whole-body' approach to the problem.

Tinnitus

This disturbing and widespread problem involves persistent buzzing, hissing, ringing or roaring noises in one or both ears. It does not always affect the hearing, although many tinnitus sufferers also have faulty hearing. Many of us have experienced temporary tinnitus, perhaps following a blow to the head or being too close to a shotgun blast or even attending a live pop concert! Fortunately the ears usually recover within 24 hours. The victims of chronic tinnitus may, however, suffer symptoms without a break for months or years. Apart from the usual tranquillizers and antidepressants, the orthodox medical treatment consists of 'maskers' that attempt to cover up the noises. This is only partly successful for the maskers themselves can be irritating.

Recent work in America has demonstrated that tinnitus is frequently caused by a metabolic imbalance involving changes in blood constituents. Dr Paul Yannick of Monmouth College, USA, attributes the symptoms to an adrenal surge following a sudden drop in the blood sugar level.[41] This can lead to a constriction of the minute and sensitive blood vesels within the ears, the ears cannot function correctly and the symptoms of tinnitus develop. This stressful effect on the blood flow to the ears may lead to a reduction in the availability of certain nutrients, in particular vitamin A, the B vitamins, zinc and chromium. (It has been found that the normal concentration of vitamin A in the inner ear may be ten times that of other tissues.)[41]

CASE HISTORY

Terry, a 32-year-old factory worker, had suffered from tinnitus (whistling in both ears), headaches, fatigue and photophobia (light sensitivity) for six years. His treatment had consisted of anti-depressant drugs and chiropractic treatment to the spine and neck. His hair mineral analysis showed low levels of chromium, magnesium, manganese, potassium and zinc. The six-hour glucose tolerance test showed a fasting level of 4mmol/litre, falling to 2.3mmol/litre during the test. His mother was an asthma sufferer and both his children had hay-fever. As a shift worker, his diet was erratic and unsuitable, consisting of toast for breakfast, sandwiches for lunch and often a take-away for dinner. He ate six to eight packets of crisps daily, several chocolate bars, and drank 12 to 15 sweet coffees every 24 hours.

Terry was prescribed a course of acupuncture to balance the energy associated with the ears. His diet was altered to reduce the starch and sugar. He was advised to take a multi-mineral with additional chromium and zinc and a B-complex formula. Beta carotene was also prescribed.

The anti-depressants were reduced over a period of two months, and after four months Terry became symptom-free.

Deafness

The imbalance caused by sudden falls in the blood sugar level, namely stress with a resulting adrenal overstimulation, also play an important role in functional deafness. Hearing loss can lead to further stress and a vicious circle may develop that perhaps only correct nutrition can relieve. Low blood sugar has been linked to raised levels of cholesterol and triglyceride in the blood (pages 79-80) and potassium deficiency with sodium excess. Dr Yannick believes that a high cholesterol or triglyceride level reduces the supply of oxygen to the inner ear. A low potassium-high sodium ratio can lead to a biochemical imbalance in the body's fluid levels.

If either of these conditions develops the hearing can be impaired. The ears, like the eyes, are very sensitive to changes within the blood constituents. Many hearing problems have a metabolic or functional basis rather than a structural cause, and an awareness of the influence of correct nutrition on the ears is of great importance.

Fatigue

One of the most common symptoms occurring in hypoglycaemia is fatigue. Glucose and its derivatives provide fuel to the nerve cells. It follows, therefore, that if the fuel is in short supply, the available energy must be reduced. Exhaustion is difficult to treat because there are so many causes. These include:

1. *Stress*. Stress can be likened to a stationary car. If you apply the choke or put your foot on the throttle the engine increases revs and uses fuel, but it does not move. In a like manner, the stressful individual may exhaust himself by simply sitting and worrying. Stress causes the adrenal glands to operate the 'fight or flight' mechanism. This may be very necessary in primitive, natural environments, but can be destructive and fatiguing on a daily

basis, as often occurs in civilized society.

2. *Overwork*. I am often amazed at the number of hours a day many people work, although this particularly applies to the self-employed, but also there are many who 'moonlight', e.g. they have two jobs involving a 12 to 16 hour day. Unfortunately, those who work hard and long often miss holidays and have erratic meal times. Not surprisingly their body cannot stand the pace and fatigue develops.

3. *Insomnia*. When confronted with a patient with fatigue, the first question must be 'Do you sleep well?' Insufficient sleep night after night, for whatever reason, must lead to extreme fatigue. Even when the diet is perfect and there is no undue stress, insufficient sleep is a prime cause of fatigue. Individual sleep requirements vary enormously – some of us can manage with five hours, others may need nine or ten hours.

4. *Smoking and drinking*. There is little need to repeat what has been said in previous chapters as both habits are destructive and energy-sapping. Faulty nutrition and low blood sugar are one of the main causes of fatigue. Nutritional deficiencies and deficiency of the blood itself can contribute to low energy.

Dr Williams has found that fatigue can result from individual requirements for vitamins and minerals far in excess of accepted normal requirements.[31] If these requirements are not met with supplements to the diet, then that person may become extremely tired. There is no quick answer to the person who is constantly tired. Elimination of the foregoing list is a first step to solving the problem. It should be remembered, however, that fatigue is a symptom of many serious illnesses requiring detailed and specific tests, and these include:

Diabetes	Leukaemia
Arthritis	Acute and chronic infections
Cancer	Drug side effects
Anaemia	Nervous disorders
Thyroid imbalance	Absorption problems
Heart conditions	TB
Malnutrition	Kidney disease

ME (Myalgic Encephalomyelitis) or Post-viral Fatigue Syndrome

Low blood sugar can produce many symptoms of physical and mental stress that may develop into other illnesses. These include diabetes, depression, migraine asthma etc. A very common symptom, however, is fatigue, and many patients with ME or PVFS can confirm that their early symptoms were often typical of low blood sugar. As glucose is the main body fuel and low blood sugar is usually associated with physical and mental fatigue, I always check ME patients for hypoglycaemia and look very carefully at their past health and eating habits.

This chapter has, I hope, shown the diversity of diseases and symptoms that can be caused or influenced by hypoglycaemia. All the conditions discussed can be due to other causes. It is worth remembering, however, that there is, in every instance, a link with hypoglycaemia which has been proved, and evidence is available to show that the dietary approach so essential in hypoglycaemia has provided symptom relief – often in many cases where other treatment has failed.

11

DIAGNOSIS

As hypoglycaemia masquerades as so many different conditions and can create such a diversity of symptoms, it is not
always easy to diagnose. For this reason, and others which
will be discussed later, it is not wise to diagnose and treat
hypoglycaemia without professional help. Hypoglycaemia
mimics very many serious diseases, and it is therefore essential that the more serious causes of hypoglycaemic symptoms
should be ruled out.

The clinical diagnosis of hypoglycaemia falls into several
stages.

Family History

Although this subject has been briefly touched upon in other
parts of the book, I would like to show, with examples, just
how hypoglycaemia conditions can pass from generation to
generation. It follows that detailed evaluation of a person's
family health is of considerable diagnostic value.

In Table 1 (see page 24) you will see the family history
of 50 patients with confirmed reactive hypoglycaemia (as
proved by a six-hour glucose tolerance test). These have

been selected as typical low blood sugar problems and you will see that the characteristic symptoms associated with hypoglycaemia pass through each family. The majority of patients with a positive glucose tolerance test result tend to show a previous history in their family of either asthma, migraine, hay fever, diabetes, epilepsy or depression, etc.

Present Symptoms

As we know, the symptoms of hypoglycaemia can be misleading to the diagnostician: often of more significance than a list of symptoms is the pattern of cause and the time of onset of the symptoms. One patient, Mr A, may experience headaches when reading or watching television, while another patient, Mr B, may develop headaches only in the early morning or when he drinks certain types of wine. In the case of Mr A, he may well have eye strain, but Mr B could be a subject for hypoglycaemia.

Fatigue at the end of the day may suggest overwork, anaemia or a variety of causes. Fatigue on rising which improves towards the end of the day is a strong clue to a possible diagnosis of hypoglycaemia. A subjective evaluation is never easy, for unless one is very familiar with the pattern of hypoglycaemic symptoms, it is very difficult to diagnose one's own problems.

One of the chief characteristics of hypoglycaemia sufferers is the combination of physical and mental symptoms coupled with considerable variation in the symptoms. At times the patient may feel on top of the world, and at other times he may feel exhausted and depressed for no apparent reason. Remember, we are not dealing with a predictable organic disease such as overactive thyroid or anaemia, but an imbalance in the nervous, circulatory, digestive and endocrine systems. Therefore, any symptoms are the expression of a great number of interrelating and fluctuating factors. These factors are influenced by diet, emotion, menstruation, time of day, stress and fatigue, and other factors already mentioned.

Past Health

No illness suddenly arrives. There are always changes in the body before the symptoms become apparent to the patient. With hypoglycaemia the early symptoms are usually vague and difficult to identify. The commonest symptoms are fatigue associated with a dulling of concentration, irritability and mild anxiety or depression, thick-headedness on wakening and a distinct loss of zest before mid-morning. The latter symptoms may include transitory feelings of panic or breathlessness with cold sweating and headaches often accompanied by a craving for something sweet. These early symptoms are often diagnosed as being due to overwork, stress or nerves. The usual sedatives and relaxants are prescribed, but if symptoms are due to hypoglycaemia any relief will be only temporary. The fatigue will still be there and often without overwork, and the anxiety will persist often without any known stress. It is unfortunate that many hypoglycaemic patients suffer their symptoms with a false diagnosis, for years classified by doctors and family as neurotic when, in fact, the cause of their symptoms is physiological and not psychological.

When looking into a past history, there is often a history of symptoms that show promise of future hypoglycaemia. These include hepatitis, jaundice, morning sickness with pregnancy, biliousness and intolerance of fats, and a history of gall bladder trouble. The role of the body's early warning system is to indicate the development of a biochemical imbalance or damage of some kind. If the early symptoms of hypoglycaemia are accurately diagnosed before the migraines, epilepsies and diabetes develop, a great deal of pain and distress may be avoided.

Dietary Habits

Faulty nutrition can be said to be the single most important cause of hypoglycaemia. The modern diet with its high sugar content, refined starches, artificial additives, and with taste and appearance taking commercial priority over nutritional value, offers the perfect formula for causing blood sugar imbalances. If we also consider the modern habits of snack-meals, frequent coffees and the excessive use of drugs, alcohol and tobacco, it is no surprise that the incidence of high and low blood sugar conditions is increasing at an alarming rate.

As poor diet is a key factor in the cause and maintenance of hypoglycaemia, it is obviously an important clue in the diagnosis of this problem. I find in practice that most hypo-glycaemic sufferers have characteristic dietary habits which provide important leads to the cause of their symptoms. It must be remembered that, for the hypoglycaemic, meals are not simply a question of choice, for the pattern of meals and type of food is strongly influenced by the underlying low blood sugar. Sugary foods and drink, caffeine-rich or alcohol-rich drinks all provide temporary relief to the symptoms of hypoglycaemia. Not surprisingly, the diet reflects this and is high in these items. Often there may be cravings for sweet food, etc. far in excess of normal consumption and, as discussed in Chapter 10, most alcoholics and tobacco addicts are hypoglycaemic.

One of the most significant clues is the sugar intake – two

to three teaspoonsful in either tea or coffee is not unusual. Because hypoglycaemia is linked to the appetite, a frequent symptom is hunger, not the type of hunger that most of us experience if we miss a meal, but a ravenous hunger, very often a craving for a certain type of food. Conversely, the hypoglycaemic patient, because of the symptoms produced by his condition, cannot face food. This usually occurs at breakfast time as the blood sugar drops overnight. The thought of breakfast can make a person with hypoglycaemia almost physically sick. Usually a coffee or cigarette starts the day, and the inevitable 'high' provided by the caffeine produces a mid-morning 'low' as the blood sugar drops again. So the day consists of small frequent 'shots' of sugar or caffeine to keep the energy level and the concentration in a tolerable balance.

The hypoglycaemic is a night nibbler, often waking with stomach cramp, indigestion or just hunger, usually around 3 a.m. to 5 a.m. when the blood sugar has sunk to a low level.

The two diets listed below are not only typical diets of those who become hypoglycaemic, but the actual diets of two patients seen in my practice. Every characteristic of the hypoglycaemic's eating habits can be seen here and, although in each case a glucose tolerance test was requested, the two patients were, not surprisingly, diagnosed as hypoglycaemic.

EXAMPLE 1

Breakfast Cereal with sugar and milk. 4–5 cups of tea – 1 teaspoonful of sugar in each cup.

11 a.m. Tea with a biscuit or cake.

Lunch Sandwich with tea and biscuit.

4 p.m. Cake with tea.

Dinner Meat and vegetables with sweet dessert. Cup of tea.

Supper Crackers, cheese, biscuits and tea.

— Tea – 12–14 cups daily.
— Coffee – rarely.
— Cigarettes – 20–30 a day.
— Sweets and chocolate – 4–6oz (100–175g) a day.

EXAMPLE 2

Breakfast   2 coffees with 2½ teaspoonsful of sugar in each.
11 a.m.   Coffee with biscuits.
Lunch   Toast with egg or cheese. 2 coffees.
4.30 p.m.   Cake with coffee.
Dinner   Meat and vegetables with coffee.
Supper   Cake with coffee.

— Tea – nil.
— Coffee – 8–10 cups daily.
— Cigarettes – 10–12 a day.
— Sweets and chocolates – 2oz (50g) a day approximately.

Physical Examination

There is only one physical sign of hypoglycaemia – a tenderness over the pancreas in the left upper quadrant of the abdomen, often extending as low as the umbilicus. This tenderness is felt just below the rib, or at times round the side of the rib cage. It is due to pancreatic sensitivity which, as we know, is due to hyperinsulinism. In practice I find that if I press most patients' abdomens hard enough they are tender in many places. The test is therefore to press with the same gentle pressure all over the stomach, liver and pancreas areas and then ask the patient, 'Which is the most tender?' The fingers encounter a feeling of tightness, or even hardness, accompanying the discomfort. This sign usually disappears as treatment progresses, and provides confirmation that the situation is normalizing.

Although the patient's weight, colouring, blood pressure, etc. are all significant in hypoglycaemia, they are all influenced by many other disorders and are therefore not of special value in diagnosing hypoglycaemia.

The Six-hour Glucose Tolerance Test

This test is the most reliable test for reactive hypoglycaemia and is usually referred to as the GTT. The customary test of two hours is frequently used, and although it may be sufficient for a diagnosis of diabetes, it is virtually valueless as a means of establishing reactive hypoglycaemia, since the important overswing invariably occurs after more than two hours. The GTT is only a valid diagnostic tool if the following conditions are met:

1. It is combined with a physical examination.

2. The test is preceded by noting down a detailed case history.

3. The patient has described and listed his own diet and symptoms.

4. The patient's reactions and symptoms during the test are noted and timed.

5. The glucose dosage and timing of blood sample taking is standardized for every test.

6. No dramatic changes have recently been made to the diet.

7. The physician is fully aware of any drugs being taken by the patient.

It must be remembered that some hypoglycaemics do not show any symptoms, while other patients show pronounced hypoglycaemic symptoms with a normal blood sugar level. Hence the need to standardize the test procedures and to know each patient as thoroughly as possible before the test.

TEST PROCEDURE

The patient is requested to undergo a 14-hour fast, (water only permitted), and to attend the surgery at 9.00 a.m. The fast is no great hardship as only breakfast is missed. Obviously it is important that no food or drink (except water) is taken until the test is completed at 3.30 p.m. As cigarettes and certain drugs influence the blood sugar it is essential not to smoke during the test, and patients are requested to provide information at least a week before the test on their current medical treatment.

During the course of the test, seven small blood samples are taken from the veins of the arm. (Only 1ml of whole blood being required per sample.) The first sample, taken at 9.15 a.m., shows the level of fasting blood sugar (FBS), and is followed at 9.30 a.m. by the drinking of 50g (2 oz) of soluble glucose. The remaining six samples are then taken to monitor the effects of the glucose on the patient's blood sugar level. The amount of glucose used in the GTT can vary, 100g (4 oz) being the usual test dose in America. This higher dose can occasionally make the more sensitive patients nauseous or faint, and is not normally used in this country. (There is no available evidence to suggest that 100g (4 oz) improves diagnostic accuracy.)

The blood sugar level is constantly changing, even with seven samples taken in six hours, one obtains only a guide to the dynamics of blood glucose activities. For this reason, the highest reading may in fact lie *between* two samples. If I suspect that this has occurred and the speed of the patient's insulin response has been so rapid that the GTT has not confirmed diagnosis – a repeat test is requested. This is a shorter version, also using 50g (2 oz) of glucose but with a sample taken very 15 minutes over a 1½-hour period. In this way the all-important upper figure is more precisely assessed.

The sample times are obviously at the convenience of the practitioner. I find the following schedule most suitable.

Patient arrives	9.00 a.m.
Sample 1. FBS taken	9.15 a.m.
50g glucose taken	9.30 a.m.
Sample 2.	10.00 a.m.
Sample 3.	10.30 a.m.
Sample 4.	11.30 p.m.
Sample 5.	12.30 p.m.
Sample 6.	2.00 p.m.
Sample 7.	3.30 p.m.

This means that the samples are taken at the following times *after* drinking the glucose.

Sample 2.	½ hour
Sample 3.	1 hour
Sample 4.	2 hours
Sample 5.	3 hours
Sample 6.	4½ hours
Sample 7.	6 hours

The patient is encouraged to rest during the test as exercise can influence the blood sugar level. Restroom facilities are available and most patients under test have a little doze, read or knit.

As many patients do not feel very alert after the completion of the test, they are advised to arrange for a 'chauffeur' (relative or neighbour) to drive them home. It is also sensible to have a small protein snack as soon as possible after completion of the test. The results usually return from the laboratory within 48 hours.

Symptoms Produced by the GTT

The symptoms that arise during the test, and the timing of the onset of these symptoms are both of diagnostic value.

When the glucose readings are explained to the patient on his/her next visit, it is always interesting to note that the symptoms experienced during the test, (e.g. nausea, headache, stomach pains, lethargy, dizziness), usually developed as the blood sugar fell. The majority of patients are quite impressed to learn that their symptoms often attributed to stress or imagination can be reproduced by the simple method of taking a glucose drink. For them, this confirms the diagnosis of hypoglycaemia in a far more tangible way than could a set of blood test results. This clinical confirmation of a puzzling condition is often very reassuring to the patient. Where patients have a long-term condition, however, e.g. migraine, asthma, etc. the symptoms do not always reproduce during the six-hour test. I have seen GTT results showing profound low blood sugar changes, yet the patient has felt quite well during the testing. This apparent lack of reaction to the changes that occur during the test may be explained in two ways.

1. The patient's metabolism has adjusted to the condition over many years, usually as a result of glandular compensation, and although symptoms still exist 50g of glucose is

not sufficient to reproduce these symptoms during the test, although the glucose *is* sufficient to produce the characteristic drop in the blood sugar level.

2. There is frequently a delayed symptom response to the test and it is always well to advise patients that they may feel rather poorly the next day.

GTT Results

This valuable test can establish a diagnosis of diabetes or hypoglycaemia. Although the medical orthodox view holds that reactive hypoglycaemia is a rare condition, the evidence points to the contrary. I have found that out of 210 patients selected and tested with a six-hour GTT, 92% showed clearly defined reactive hypoglycaemia.

Since Seale Harris first described hypoglycaemia in 1924, no one generally accepted guideline defining this condition has been agreed upon. The GTT is open to various interpretations, depending on the doctor's view of what constitutes the 'normal'. (As with many types of measurement used in medicine, the figures for the average patient cannot necessarily be taken as the normal!)

Dr Harris has stated, that in his view a diagnosis of hypoglycaemia is justified if the GTT shows a blood sugar reading *below* the commonly accepted lower limit 4-6mmol/litre. This, he insisted, must be supported by the reproduction of hypoglycaemic symptoms during the course of the test. Over the intervening years the required lower limit, below which hypoglycaemia could be established, has been reduced to 2mmol/litre.

This rather rigid criterion for diagnosis has fortunately been modified in recent years, with the general recognition that each GTT result should be assessed in relation to the patient. An individual's response to the glucose drink should be observed in terms of speed of absorption, and speed of insulin response.

A patient may have pronounced symptoms of hypoglycaemia yet shows a set of glucose readings, all of which are within 'normal' limits. Close attention to symptoms before and during the GTT is of greater diagnostic value than slavish adherence to a set of normal ranges.

I have seen patients experience distressing symptoms of hypoglycaemia when their blood sugar has fallen during a GTT from 8mmol/litre to 4mmol/litre, the symptoms being caused not by the *level* of glucose but by the inappropriate *speed* of the fall. A fall in excess of 1.5mmol/litre per hour is significant!

It may be of value to discuss the *normal* GTT result, before going further, and the manner in which the result is presented (Table 7).

When the glucose has been taken by the patient, the blood sugar rises (Samples 2 and 3). As the glucose is absorbed, insulin is automatically released to control the rising blood sugar. With a normal insulin response, only an optimum amount of insulin is released allowing the blood sugar level to fall into the patient's fasting level (Sample 7).

The results are plotted on a graph and a glucose tolerance curve is produced. Examples of typical curves are shown below (Figures 5-14). One learns to recognize different types of curves, for the configuration of a curve is diagnostically as important as the actual figures producing it.

Diagnosis Using the GTT

When presented with a set of figures for a GTT the first step

Table 7 Normal Six-hour GTT Result

Sample	Interval from 0 in hours	Time	Result in mmol/litre
1	0 (F.B.S.)	9.15 a.m.	4.4
	(50 g glucose solution)	(9.30 a.m.)	
2	½	10.00 a.m.	6.6
3	1	10.30 a.m.	5.3
4	2	11.30 a.m.	4.7
5	3	12.30 p.m.	4.1
6	4½	2.00 p.m.	4.2
7	6	3.30 p.m.	4.4

is to look for a possible diabetic component. A fasting level in excess of 8mmol/litre is strongly suggestive of diabetes, but some diabetics can have a fasting level under 6mmol/litre. For this reason an assessment of the sum of the first four results obtained in the GTT is recommended by Dr Danowski of Pittsburgh,[27] as a more reliable method of identifying diabetes. If the *total* for the four samples is between 28–44 mmol/litre, diabetes is suspected; if *over* 44mmol/litre, diabetes is positively confirmed.

There are many different types of GTT curves, for the dynamics of the blood sugar level is expressed in many ways. As stated, the actual level of blood sugar is related to symptoms during the test, but even more important is, perhaps, the speed at which the blood sugar responds to the insulin. A drop of from 6.5mmol/litre to 3.5mmol/litre in one hour may be more significant than a drop from 6.5mmol/litre to 2.5mmol/litre in two hours. The time taken for the sugar to return to a normal level (usually called the 'recovery'), and how long it remains at a low level, are also important diagnostic clues. For example, a fall to 2.5mmol/litre with a rapid recovery to normal may be less significant than a fall to

3.5mmol/litre that stays at this level for two to three hours before recovery.

It is very unusual to find any two GTT curves that are alike. So called 'normal' values are based on population averages and may not reflect what is normal for the patient being tested.

Some disagreement surrounds the value of interpreting the 'fall' in blood sugar during the test. This represents the difference between the initial fasting level, and the lowest figure to which the blood sugar drops during the test. Atkins[27] considers a 1.5mmol/litre drop essential before a conclusive diagnosis of hypoglycaemia can be given, whilst Fredericks[42] find that a drop of between 0.5-1mmol/litre is sufficient. Other authorities (e.g. Somgyi) have set the figures of 0.25-0.5mmol/litre as diagnostically significant. These figures are, however, meaningful only within the context of symptoms arising during the test and an individual's reaction to the 50g (2 oz) of glucose. I find in practice that as little as a 0.5mmol/litre fall can be associated with hypoglycaemic symptoms.

To conclude this description of GTT, it may be worth quoting Carlton Fredericks,[42] an authority on many aspects of nutrition. He states that 'When blood sugar drops as little as 0.25mmol/litre below the *normal for the patient*, a profound glandular compensation may start.'

In his view, no practitioner should disregard a blood sugar reading that is 'only a few points below normal' and if there is doubt, a diagnosis of hypoglycaemia with correct treatment should be considered.

The following are some typical blood sugar curves.

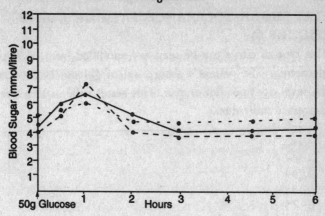

Figure 5 Normal blood sugar curves

NORMAL BLOOD SUGAR CURVES (FIGURE 5)

These curves are of healthy individuals. The fasting test (the first reading) varies, but at no time during the six hours does the blood sugar fall much below the fasting level.

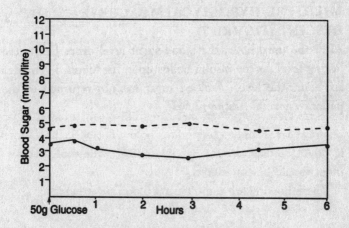

Figure 6 Flat sugar-tolerance fatigue curve

FLAT SUGAR-TOLERANCE 'FATIGUE' CURVE (FIGURE 6)

This type of curve can be seen as a modified form of hypoglycaemia. The patient's absorption of glucose is poor and the level does not fall or rise. This result reflects a fatigued, depressed individual.

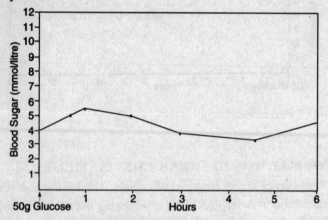

Figure 7 Mild pre-hypoglycaemic curve (slow descent)

MILD, PRE-HYPOGLYCAEMIC CURVE – SLOW DESCENT (FIGURE 7)

After the third hour, the blood sugar level drops below the fasting level, as the insulin builds up in the blood. Even after six hours the level of blood sugar has not returned to the patient's normal (fasting) level.

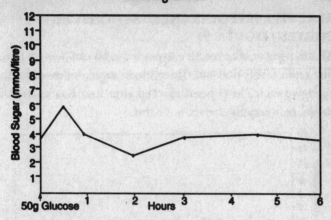

Figure 8 Mild Hypoglycaemic curve (rapid descent)

MILD HYPOGLYCAEMIA – RAPID DESCENT (FIGURE 8)

Although there is not a great difference between the fasting level and the lowest point reached, the *speed* of descent suggests rapid and excessive insulin reaction.

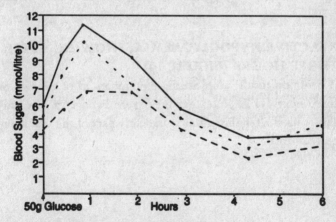

Figure 9 Reactive hypoglycaemia (typical curves)

REACTIVE HYPOGLYCAEMIA – TYPICAL CURVES (FIGURE 9)

All the signs of true reactive hypoglycaemia can be seen here. The rapid absorption and rise in blood sugar; followed by the hypoglycaemic 'low' point reached after four hours, and the partial recovery by the six-hour test.

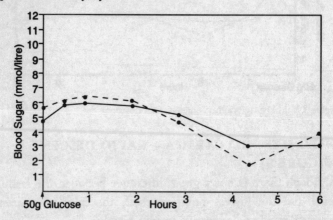

Figure 10 Reactive hypoglycaemia showing after three hours (typical curve)

REACTIVE HYPOGLYCAEMIA, SHOWING AFTER THREE HOURS (FIGURE 10)

A common result, emphasizing the limitations of the two or three hour GTT. Note that the severe hypoglycaemia only shows itself after three hours; the early part of the test being quite normal.

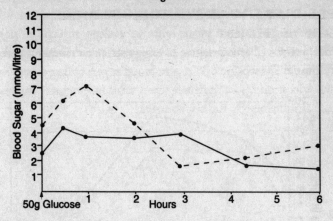

Figure 11 Reactive hypoglycaemia (severe curves)

REACTIVE HYPOGLYCAEMIA – SEVERE CURVES (FIGURE 11)

Often a low fasting level with a further drop into very low readings. Patients with symptoms during the test are usually found to have this type of severe curve.

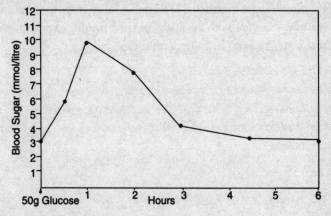

Figure 12 Pre-diabetic curve

PRE-DIABETIC CURVE (FIGURE 12)

Steep rise in blood sugar with very slow return to normal level. Characteristics of sluggish pre-diabetic insulin response.

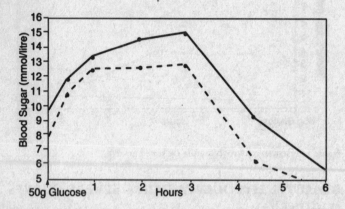

Figure 13 Dysinsulinism

DYSINSULINISM (FIGURE 13)

The blood sugar paradox. Delayed insulin response causing high blood sugar, with an inappropriate insulin excess in the third hour, causing hypoglycaemic-type fall.

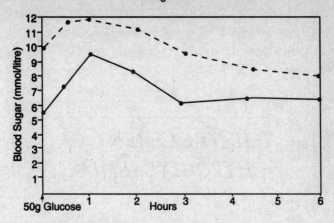

Figure 14 Diabetic curve

DIABETIC CURVE (FIGURE 14)
Typical diabetic curves, high fasting levels and insufficient insulin to normalize blood sugar level.

12

THE TREATMENT OF HYPOGLYCAEMIA

I wish that I could state that there is *one* diet recommended by the various 'experts' for treating reactive hypoglycaemia. Regrettably this is not the case, as most of the writers and specialists seem to want to promote their own diet. This should seem to offer a welcome variety to the reader and choice to the patient; unfortunately, it causes only confusion. This habit occurs mainly because of the common habit of most writers on hypoglycaemia of recommending their own treatment programme at the expense of other treatments, frequently stating that the other people's diets and treatment are useless or even dangerous.

Dietary Requirements[67]

There are, however, certain principles or requirements which must be met if a diet for hypoglycaemia is to be effective. These can be listed as follows:

1. Total carbohydrate consumption must be reduced, and refined (quickly absorbed) carbohydrates, including sugar, chocolate, sweets etc. must be *avoided*.

2. There should be five or six small meals daily.

3. The diet should be relatively high in fat and protein which should be spread over the day.

4. The total calorie content of the diet should be around 2,500 calories.

5. The diet should include a substantial breakfast and supper, to be taken as early and as late as possible.

6. Stimulants that will increase and subsequently lower the blood sugar (owing to hyperinsulinism) must be avoided. These include alcohol, tobacco and caffeine.

Although I do not agree with some of the diets recommended by American authors, it may be of interest to discuss briefly the various dietary approaches to hypoglycaemia. (One problem with reading too many American publications on hypoglycaemia is that the American diet is somewhat different from the English diet. We rarely come across eggplant, kohlrabi or collards on a British shopping list!)

THE SEALE HARRIS DIET (HIGH FAT AND HIGH PROTEIN)

Still recommended by many doctors and writers, this diet was described by Dr Harris in his first paper on hypoglycaemia,[9] and has a strong supporter in Dr Abrahamson.[18]

The Harris diet is as follows:

On rising   100ml (4 fl oz) of orange juice

Breakfast   1 fruit, with or without cream – no sugar.
    1 serving of cereal with cream – no sugar.
    1 egg and, if desired, 2 or 3 slices of bacon.

1 slice of bread or toast with butter (liberally spread).
Caffeine-free coffee, or very weak tea — no sugar.

2 hours after 75ml (3 fl oz) of orange juice or 100ml
breakfast (4 fl oz) of tomato juice.

3 hours after 1 glass of milk.
breakfast

Lunch Soup (cold or jellied chicken or beef *consommé*)
or tomato juice.
225g(8 oz) vegetables.
1 large portion of meat, poultry or fish.
1 slice of bread or toast.
Fruit with cream.

3 hours after 1 glass of milk.
lunch

1 hour before 75 ml (3 fl oz) of orange juice or 100ml
dinner (4 fl oz) of tomato juice

Dinner One meat 'substitute' — egg, cheese or fish.
Salad — large serving of lettuce, coleslaw, tomato, *or*
Waldorf salad with mayonnaise or French dressing.
1 portion of vegetables.
1 slice of bread with plenty of butter.
Fruit.

2-3 hours 1 glass of milk.
after dinner

Every 2 100ml (4 fl oz) of orange or tomato juice.
hours until
bed-time

It has been used as a basis for many of the diets prescribed for hypoglycaemia, and we owe a great deal to Dr Harris for his observations almost 60 years ago.

The Airola Diet

(Low Animal Protein – High Natural Carbohydrate)
The American author, Dr Paavo Airola, has evolved a diet that contains (in order of importance):

1. Grains, seeds and nuts

2. Vegetables

3. Fruit

Dr Airola[43] claims that raw and sprouted grains and seeds should be the main protein source, animal proteins being kept to a minimum. All seeds and nuts are eaten fresh and raw, and cereals are permitted provided they are eaten in their 'whole' state and not refined. Millet is especially recommended. He recommends that meat be eaten on a weekly basis, if at all. The diet is as follows:

7 *a.m.*   Glass of fruit juice. Sweet juices must be diluted with water 50/50.

8 *a.m.*   BREAKFAST. Nuts, seeds, fruit, yogurt, cottage cheese. OR, cooked cereal with oil and raw milk.

10 *a.m.*   Snack – a few nuts, or glass of yoghurt, or piece of fruit.

12 *noon*   Glass of fresh juice.

1 p.m.　　　LUNCH. Cooked cereal: buckwheat, millet, etc. with oil and milk, if not eaten for breakfast, OR, fruit or vegetable salad with yogurt and 2 slices of wholewheat bread with cheese and butter.

3 p.m.　　　Glass of juice or kefir with 2 tablespoonsful of yeast.

5 p.m.　　　Glass of fresh vegetable juice.

6 p.m.　　　DINNER. Vegetable salad with cooked vegetable dish of: beans, tortillas, yams, green beans, baked potatoes, etc. Slice or two of wholewheat bread. Cottage cheese, yogurt. Animal protein if desired.

8 p.m.　　　Glass of milk or yogurt with 1 or 2 tablespoonsful of brewer's yeast.

High Protein Diet

Perhaps the commonest dietary treatment of hypoglycaemia is simply to instruct patients to avoid all forms of refined starch and eat lots of protein and fat. Fredericks advocates a daily consumption of 300-75g (11-13oz) of meat. This should be in the form of six meals with meat or 'meat substitute' (e.g. cheese) at every meal.

Common Factors

Clearly these various diets for hypoglycaemia are all quite different; yet in each case the diet seems to work, and evidence is available to confirm the efficiency of each regime. This paradox is probably due to certain common factors in the diets, namely, the avoidance of refined starch and the insistence upon five or six regular meals.

Diets work only if the patient is prepared to follow them for a prescribed period of time. With the hypoglycaemic diet it is essential to maintain the diet for an initial period of eight to twelve weeks. It follows that any diet must fulfil these requirements:

1. It should not contain expensive or exotic food (e.g. fillet steak daily).

2. Many patients work full time and cannot prepare elaborate dishes; the meals must be simple, particularly as there are four to six meals per day.

3. The diet should not be too unsociable and too different from the average diet. Otherwise, I have found that patients are too easily tempted to 'stray' off the recommended foods.

4. The meals should be tasty and enjoyable.

5. Since many hypoglycaemics are overweight (especially the ladies), and very conscious of extra pounds, the diet should not cause one to put on weight.

6. Finally, and perhaps most obvious, the diet must work. Only by feeling better will a patient continue to follow a strict diet, week after week.

Although I frequently draw up individual diets for patients, they are usually based on a standard diet as set out below:

Recommended Diet

The standard diet that I use is as follows:

On rising   Medium orange, ½ grapefruit or 100ml (4 fl oz) fruit juice or cup of beverage or milk.

Breakfast   Fruit or 100ml (4 fl oz) fruit juice.
1 egg, with or without 2 slices of ham or bacon, or cheese or fish dish.
1 slice of wholewheat bread or toast, with plenty of butter.
Milk or beverage.

2 hours after   100ml (4 fl oz) fruit juice.
breakfast

Lunch   Meat, fish, cheese or eggs with salad – large serving of lettuce or tomato with mayonnaise or French dressing.
Vegetables if desired.
1 slice of wholewheat bread, toast or crisp-bread with plenty of butter.

3 hours after   100ml (4 fl oz) milk
lunch

1 hour before   100ml (4 fl oz) fruit juice.
dinner

Dinner   Soup, if desired (not thickened with flour).
Vegetables.
Meat, fish or poultry.
1 slice of wholewheat bread, if desired.
Dessert (fruit – fresh, stewed or baked) and beverage.

Every 2 hours Small handful of nuts (unsalted).
until bed-time

Supper   Crispbread with cottage cheese or *pâté*, with
  butter. Beverage or milk.

NOTES

Live fresh yogurt or goat's milk is preferred to cow's milk.
Where butter is mentioned, vegetable margarine may be
substituted. If the dairy products are unacceptable, owing
to catarrh or migraine or asthma, substitute soya milk, plant
milk or other non-animal products. IT IS ADVISABLE TO
AVOID THE USE OF SYNTHETIC SUGAR SUBSTITUTES.

Allowable Food and Drink

VEGETABLES

Asparagus, beets, broccoli, brussels, lettuce, mushrooms,
nuts, cabbage, cauliflower, carrots, celery, sweetcorn,
cucumber, beans, onions, peas, radishes, sauerkraut, tomatoes, turnips, swede, parsnips and any other vegetables not
on the 'avoid' list.

FRUIT

Apples, apricots, strawberries, raspberries, blackberries,
grapefruit, melon, oranges, peaches, pears, pineapple,
tangerines, avocados. May be cooked or raw with or without
cream, but *without* sugar.

JUICE

Any unsweetened fruit or vegetable juice, except grape juice
or prune juice. *Avoid* tinned fruit juice unless pure.

BEVERAGES
Decaffeinated coffee or herb teas.

DESSERTS
Fruit — fresh, stewed or baked.

SALT
Use sea salt in moderation, or low sodium salt.

AVOID ABSOLUTELY
Any foods not mentioned on the diet and, in particular, *sugar*; chocolate and other sweets etc., such as cake, pie, pastries, sweet custards, puddings, ice-cream; salted nuts; and *all cereal products*; diabetic foods; syrup; molasses; and honey. Avoid ordinary coffee; tea, alcohol; soft drinks; beverages containing caffeine; tobacco; potatoes; rice; grapes; raisins; plums; figs; dates; bananas; spaghetti, macaroni and noodles. THESE DIETS SHOULD ONLY BE USED UNDER THE DIRECT AND REGULAR SUPERVISION OF A PRACTITIONER.

Why the Hypoglycaemic Diet?

When the majority of patients first encounter the diet prescribed for hypoglycaemia, they are understandably baffled by the ban on sugar. They have been given a diagnosis of low blood sugar and yet they must avoid sugar. Hypoglycaemia is the opposite of diabetes, and diabetics cannot have sugar; therefore, surely the hypoglycaemic sufferer must eat lots of sugar?

Another area of misunderstanding is the question of sugar falling when we miss meals. It has been acknowledged for many years that controlled fasting can be eliminative and rejuvenating. 'Why,' the low blood sugar patient asks, 'do I feel so ill with an overnight fast, when prolonged fasts are frequently recommended at health clinics?'

Throughout our lives we are instructed and persuaded that sugar gives us energy. Sugar, honey, glucose and molasses are names synonymous with vitality. The hypoglycaemic patient is exhausted and depressed. It can, therefore, be very confusing to be told that he will feel better if he avoids all foods and drinks that are traditionally thought to provide energy.

There are sound physiological reasons why sugar and refined carbohydrates must be avoided. Neat sugar is absorbed too quickly and the body reacts by discharging insulin into the blood. We know that hyperinsulinism is the central problem in reactive hypoglycaemia, and sugar aggravates and perpetuates this problem. Our digestive systems needs a small amount of carbohydrate in order to efficiently break down and absorb proteins and fats. This, however, can be supplied by taking non-refined carbohydrates (e.g. wholewheat bread, wholemeal cereal and the starch content in fruit and vegetables).

In the context of blood sugar balance, the colour of the sugar is irrelevant. Both brown and white sugar have the same disturbing effects. Honey's sweetness is derived chiefly from sucrose (white sugar) and molasses has similar effects. For this reason both items are barred from the diet.

Synthetic Sugar

This may be a useful point at which to mention synthetic sugars. Although, from the purely chemical viewpoint, they should not influence the insulin-glucose balance, there are two facts worth noting.

1. If one needs to follow a low blood sugar diet for several months, and possibly always avoid sweet foods, it makes dieting considerably easier if all forms of sweetness are avoided, including synthetic sweeteners (e.g. saccharine).

2. Carlton Fredericks[42] maintains that synthetic sweeteners trigger the pancreas into activity rather like a conditioned reflex. He points out that even the smell of food can stimulate the gall bladder into activity and many physical changes (e.g. allergies, migraine, etc.) can be triggered off by the smell and taste of food.

Frequency of Meals

An important characteristic of the hypoglycaemic diet is the need for frequent meals. As we know, the hypoglycaemic patient produces too much insulin in response to certain foods, and the blood sugar falls. The only way to avoid a severe drop in the blood sugar is to eat small meals at frequent intervals. Frequent snack meals of starch (e.g. sandwiches, cereal, etc.) would serve only to aggravate the problem, as all forms of carbohydrate are absorbed very quickly. Protein and fats are, however, slowly absorbed and the sensitive insulin apparatus is not triggered. Small regular meals consisting of protein or fats serve to stabilize the blood sugar, and sudden rises and falls in the glucose level are avoided.

This levelling off of the blood sugar throughout the day is extremely important, as it is the *speed* of elevation that triggers off the insulin response and not the *amount* of rise (e.g. an increase of 4mmol–6mmol/litre of sugar in the blood will produce as much pancreatic response as a rise from 10mmol–12mmol/litre). The drinks between meals prevent overeating as they serve to reduce the almost unbearable craving for food so characteristic of hypoglycaemia. The milk drinks have the job of 'topping up' between meals, for without them the blood sugar would drop and symptoms would develop. In severe cases it may even be necessary to chew protein tablets between meals or take frequent soya-based protein drinks.

Proteins

I find the concept of a high protein diet unacceptable and unnecessary, and prefer to talk in terms of a 'protein-spread' diet. This means simply, normal protein consumption with plenty of variety in choice of protein sources, but to have the protein at least four times daily. As I have already said, proteins and fats are absorbed slowly and do not upset the insulin-glucose ratio.

Fat is recommended in the diet as it depresses pancreatic activity. It should be remembered, however, that this diet is a short-term corrective programme, and it may be unwise to consume the amount of fat recommended in the diet for long periods. This particularly applies to patients with a history of heart or circulation problems, or with a high level of fat in the blood. (It is usual, if a high cholesterol or triglyceride factor is suspected, to measure these with blood tests before placing the patient on the high fat diet.)

In this context it is worth looking at the use of oils to replace solid fats in cooking. The Mediterranean Diet[63][64][65][66] with its emphasis on fowl, fish, oil and garlic combined with fresh fruit and vegetables offers an ideal basis for a satisfactory diet for the treatment of low blood sugar, without running the risk of increasing the blood fats.

PLANT PROTEINS

Perhaps the best book on the vegetarian and vegan approach to low blood sugar is *Hypoglycaemia: A Better Approach* by Paava Airola.[43] He makes the following important observation: 'Vegetable protein foods are just as good or better than animal protein. Vegetable foods which contain all eight essential amino acids (essential amino acids cannot be synthesized by the body and therefore must be present in the food we eat), are therefore complete protein foods. These include soya beans, pumpkin seeds, potatoes, peanuts, almonds, buckwheat, sunflower seeds, avocados and all green leafy vegetables. However amino acids (protein components) in eggs, milk and meat are utilized more easily and efficiently than plant protein. There is therefore a need to have plenty of variety in the plant proteins to ensure a complementary effect over each day.'

Vegetarian Diet for Low Blood Sugar[67]

On rising   1 piece of fruit *or* 100ml (4 fl oz) fresh fruit juice (50% water).

Breakfast   ONE of the following:
Sugar-free baked beans on toast.
Mushrooms or tomatoes on toast.
Vegetarian *pâté* or cheese on toast.
An egg dish.
Wholegrain cereal with milk.
Yoghurt with fresh fruit.
Drink Herb tea, decaffeinated coffee, weak China or Indian tea.

2 hours after 100ml (4 fl oz) fresh fruit juice *or* beverage
breakfast

Lunch   Mixed fresh salad with french dressing/cider vinegar/lemon juice or sugar-free mayonnaise.

Add vegetarian savoury rice, cheese, nuts or fruit as desired or eggs. One slice of wholemeal bread or Ryvita with vegetable margarine.

Drink As breakfast.

2 hours after As morning break.
lunch

Dinner   Home made soup *or* fruit.

Mixed vegetables with vegetarian savoury, can include cheese dish, stuffed peppers or tomatoes, savoury rice, mushrooms, vegetable pie or casserole, vegetarian savouries, lentil savouries, aubergines, courgettes, soya dishes, wholegrain pasta or an egg dish.

Desserts   Stewed, baked or fresh fruit *or* yoghurt *or* Ryvita with cheese.

Drink As breakfast.

Supper   (As late as possible).

Protein snack is essential.

Pâté or cheese with Ryvita or bread.

Milk or beverage to drink.

Notes   Lunch and dinner may be reversed.

It is advisable to avoid the use of sugar substitutes.

Allowable Food and Drink

VEGETABLES
Asparagus, beets, broccoli, brussels, lettuce, mushrooms, nuts, cabbage, cauliflower, carrots, celery, sweetcorn, cucumber, beans, onions, peas, radishes, sauerkraut, tom-atoes, turnips, swede, parsnips and any other vegetables not on the 'avoid' list.

FRUIT
Apples, apricots, avocados, berries, grapefruit, melons, oranges, peaches, pears, pineapple, tangerines. May be cooked or raw, *without* sugar.

JUICE
Any unsweetened fruit or vegetable juice, except grape juice or prune juice. *Avoid* tinned fruit juice unless sugar-free.

BEVERAGES
Any natural coffee substitute or decaffeinated coffee. Herb teas or weak China or Indian tea.

DESSERTS
Fruit (fresh, stewed or baked – no added sugar). Cheese. Sugar-free natural desserts or yoghurt.

ALCOHOLIC AND SOFT DRINKS
Generally best avoided, but 'slimline' sugar-free and diabetic drinks may be taken occasionally.

TOBACCO
To be avoided.

AVOID ABSOLUTELY

Any foods not mentioned on the diet, particularly sugar, chocolate and other sweets, such as cakes, pies, pastries, sweet custards, puddings, ice-cream, salted nuts, syrup, molasses and honey; caffeine – ordinary coffee, strong tea, beverages containing caffeine. THIS DIET IS TO BE USED ONLY UNDER THE DIRECT AND REGULAR SUPERVISION OF A PRACTITIONER.

Vegan Diet for Low Blood Sugar[67]

On rising   1 piece of fresh fruit *or* 4oz fresh fruit juice (50% water).

Breakfast   One of the following:
  Sugar-free baked beans on toast.
  Mushrooms or tomatoes on toast.
  Vegetarian pâté or vegan cheese on toast.
  Wholegrain cereal with soya milk.
  Drink   Herb tea, decaffeinated coffee, weak China or Indian tea.

2 hours after 4oz fresh fruit juice (50% water).
breakfast

Lunch   Mixed fresh salad with French dressing, cider vinegar, lemon juice or sugar-free mayonnaise. Add vegan savoury, rice, vegan cheese, nuts or fruit as desired. One slice of wholegrain bread or Ryvita with vegetable margarine.
  Drink   As breakfast.

2 hours after As morning break.
lunch

Dinner   Home-made soup *or* fruit.
Mixed vegetables with vegan savoury (vegan cheese dish, stuffed peppers or tomatoes, savoury rice, mushrooms, vegetable casserole, lentil savouries, aubergines, courgettes, soya dishes).

Desserts   Stewed, baked or fresh fruit (no added sugar).

Drink   As breakfast.

Supper   (As late as possible.) Protein snack is essential.
Pâté or cheese or soya milk with Ryvita or bread.

Notes   Lunch and Dinner may be reversed.
It is advisable to avoid the use of sugar substitutes.

Allowable Food and Drink

VEGETABLES
Asparagus, beets, broccoli, brussels, lettuce, mushrooms, nuts, cabbage, cauliflower, carrots, celery, sweetcorn, cucumber, beans, onions, peas, radishes, sauerkraut, tomatoes, turnips, swede, parsnips and any other vegetables not on the 'avoid' list.

FRUIT
Apples, apricots, berries, grapefruit, melons, oranges, peaches, pears, pineapple, tangerines and avocados. May be cooked or raw, *without* added sugar.

JUICE
Any unsweetened fruit or vegetable juice, except grape juice. Avoid tinned fruit or vegetable juice unless sugar-free.

BEVERAGES
Any natural coffee substitute or decaffeinated coffee. Herb teas or weak China or Indian tea.

DESSERTS
Fresh fruit (may be stewed or baked). Vegan cheese and sugar-free natural desserts.

ALCOHOLIC AND SOFT DRINKS
Generally best avoided, but 'Slimline' sugar-free and diabetic drinks may be taken occasionally.

TOBACCO
To be avoided.

AVOID ABSOLUTELY
Any foods not mentioned on the diet, particularly sugar, chocolate and other sweets, such as cakes, pies, pastries, sweet custards, puddings, ice cream, salted nuts, syrup, molasses and honey; caffeine – ordinary coffee, strong tea, beverages containing caffeine. THIS DIET IS TO BE USED ONLY UNDER THE DIRECT AND REGULAR SUPERVISION OF A PRACTITIONER.

Night-time 'Fast'

The diet requires that the patient has an early breakfast and a late supper. Both these meals should include either fat or protein. This recommendation is made to reduce the hours one spends 'fasting' throughout the night. As has been discussed many times in preceding chapters, the blood sugar normally falls to a low level between the hours of 3 a.m. and 5 a.m. The early morning asthma attack, the onset of migraine, panic feelings and anxiety, night-time raids on the pantry, etc. are all expressions of this phenomenon. By reducing the hours between dinner and breakfast, there is a good chance that the early morning crisis can be averted. The majority of people eat their last meal around 7 p.m. and have breakfast at 7 a.m. This 12-hour 'fast' is too long, and careful, regular eating throughout the day is pointless if a patient develops a hypoglycaemic episode every night.

I advise patients to eat a small protein supper prior to going to bed (10.30 p.m. to midnight) and to have a glass of milk on waking (6.30 a.m.-7.30 a.m.). If, in spite of this, the early morning symptoms persist, I have at times recommended that patients set their alarm to wake around 3 a.m. and have a small meal. This may be tedious, but, if the early morning symptoms can be suppressed for two to three weeks, it can be considered to be well worthwhile. After such a time the diet and other measures have usually normalized the insulin-glucose balance sufficiently to allow the patient to sleep through the night.

Prolonged Fasting

Patients often ask the question, 'If fasting aggravates low blood sugar, causing distressing symptoms, why is it that patients in health clinics can fast for three or four weeks and yet feel marvellous?' The answer to this is in two parts. Firstly, they do not feel 'marvellous' — at least not during the first two days. Patients undergoing a fluid-only fast almost certainly experience many symptoms of hypoglycaemia. These include headaches, irritability, nausea, dizziness and indigestion. (A true hypoglycaemic patient would, of course, experience more profound and sustained symptoms.)

Secondly, prolonged fasting does not cause a severe, progressive fall in the blood sugar. This is prevented by the process known as 'endogenous catabolism' which simply means that the body breaks down and utilizes its own fat and protein reserves. Seale Harris[9] has observed that patients who were literally starving to death owing to various forms of cancer, showed no symptoms of hypoglycaemia, the average blood sugar of the patients tested being 4.5mmol–5mmol/litre. This compensation process that occurs during fasting only begins to operate after the third or fourth day of the fast, hence the initial drop in blood sugar during the first 48 hours of the fast.

Tea, Coffee, Alcohol and Smoking

The question of coffee, tea and alcohol consumption and the smoking habit has been covered in Chapter 10. All these substances, directly or indirectly, contribute to the hypoglycaemic condition and must, therefore, be eliminated from the diet. It is particularly important to avoid the above list during the first few weeks of the diet, when the insulin response is still very sensitive. Dr Abrahamson[18] tells of patients whose hypoglycaemia was controlled by the proper diet, but who had severe blood sugar reactions when they took as little as *one* cup of coffee. Many investigators have shown that exposure to a smoky atmosphere can be virtually as harmful as smoking. For this reason the hypoglycaemic patient should avoid restaurants, theatres, parties, etc., where the atmosphere is often smoky.

Excessive Exercise

Although not detailed in the diet sheet it is important that the hypoglycaemic patient avoids excessive exercise; gentle non-competitive exercise on a little and often basis is to be preferred. (Many sufferers develop symptoms after heavy exercise, particularly migraine.)

Stress

Although stress, whether physical or mental, cannot always be avoided, it is advisable to avoid potentially stressful situations whenever possible. Stress can lead to an adrenal stimulation which in turn raises the glucose level of the blood. Where there is reactive hypoglycaemia this can produce similar symptoms to eating sugar, with all the consequences.

Supplementary Treatment

The regulation of sugar metabolism involves various glands and organs, chiefly the thyroid, pituitary and adrenal glands, and the liver and pancreas. It, therefore, follows that anything contributing to a malfunction or deficiency in these organs may also be a causative factor in hypoglycaemia.

There are certain specific substances that play an important role in sugar metabolism. When these nutrients are over- or under-supplied, the organs and glands involved in sugar metabolism may become over- or under-active. These minerals and vitamins are usually prescribed in conjunction with the corrective diet to speed up the normal activity of the sugar-regulating mechanism, and to minimize some of the unpleasant symptoms suffered by the hypoglycaemic patient.

Minerals

ZINC

There is a close relationship between zinc and insulin. Workers have shown that zinc can delay the absorption of glucose, leading, in some cases, to reactive hypoglycaemia.[44][45] It is also involved in the regulation of insulin release.[46] The usual supplementary dose is 20-30mg.

CHROMIUM

Although chromium is a trace element and present in very small amounts in our diet, it is nonetheless of considerable importance in hypoglycaemia. In 1955 it was identified as the so-called 'glucose tolerance factor', and a deficiency of this mineral has been shown to produce altered glucose tolerance. In 1968 it was observed that glucose tolerance tests showed improvement in elderly patients by the simple addition of chromium to their diet. An interesting bonus achieved by taking chromium is its effect on cholesterol control. Research has shown that chromium can produce a drop of around 14 per cent in the blood cholesterol when added in relatively small amounts to the diet.[47] A supplementary daily dosage of up to 1000mcg as chromium orotate, gluconate, aspartate or chelate is usually prescribed for the treatment of low blood sugar. Another excellent source of chromium is brewer's yeast.

MAGNESIUM AND CALCIUM

The value of calcium as a dietary supplement with particular reference to arthritis has been outlined in Chapter 7. It has a role in proper utilization of many minerals and vitamins D, A and C. The most abundant mineral in the body, it plays a part in nerve and muscle control, bone health, blood clotting and heart function. Its chief co-factors are phosphorous and magnesium. Dosage requirements vary from 500 to 1000mg taken as calcium carbonate, aspartate, chelate or gluconate. Magnesium is the main cell constituent mineral after potassium. It plays an important role in sodium, potassium and calcium distribution. It is involved in many enzyme systems and cell functions. Magnesium is usually included in supplements for low blood sugar. Its deficiency can lead to liver damage[48]. It is used to treat liver problems, heart disease, pre-menstrual syndrome, joint and muscle problems, high blood pressure, M.E., diabetes and epilepsy.

Dosage requirements should be in the ratio of one part magnesium to one to two parts calcium, usually in the form of magnesium chelate, gluconate, oxide or aspartate in dosages of 500 to 1500mg.

POTASSIUM

Large doses of potassium are of value in treating a diabetic patient who has 'hypo-ed' or when a hypoglycaemic patient experiences a low blood sugar episode (with symptoms of anxiety, palpitations, dizziness, cold sweating, etc.), 1g of soluble potassium chloride taken at this time very often quickly relieves the symptoms. The stress produced by hypoglycaemia causes large amounts of potassium to be lost in the urine, mainly owing to adrenal exhaustion. The potassium chloride quickly makes up this deficiency, raises the blood sugar level and reduces the hypoglycaemic symptoms.[50]

I find that a daily dose of 200mg of soluble potassium chloride is adequate with the 1g reserved for acute symptom reactions. (This emergency treatment is of particular benefit when dealing with nocturnal anxiety, and is safer and more effective than the usual medical prescription of glucose tablets or sedatives.)

MANGANESE

This mineral is often low in hair mineral analysis results, largely due to the current intensive farming and food processing leading to soil depletions. It plays a vital role in glucose tolerance, being essential for carbohydrate and protein metabolism. A high manganese intake reduces iron absorption, and a high level of dietary iron inhibits manganese absorption. Daily dosage is usually 10 to 20 mg as manganese chloride or chelate.

Vitamins

PANTOTHENIC ACID

Adrenal exhaustion and hypoglycaemia are very closely linked, the common factor being the frequent lack of pantothenic acid in both conditions. Research has shown that even a slight deficiency of pantothenic acid leads to a decrease in adrenal efficiency[51] with a subsequent imbalance in the sugar metabolism. Deficiency in this B vitamin also affects the insulin-glucose balance, causing the blood sugar to fall very rapidly when insulin is given.[52][53] As I have said, the speed of fall is of the utmost importance in hypoglycaemia.

THE VITAMIN B FAMILY

It is normal to prescribe a good high potency vitamin B complex with hypoglycaemia. They are of value in many areas of metabolism, aiding vitality, assisting assimilation of fats, and to some extent reducing the harmful effects of stress on the different organs and tissues. The B vitamins also serve to normalize sugar metabolism. Vitamin B_6[56] and B_{12}[55] are of special value in helping the adrenal glands, pancreas and the liver to normalize.

VITAMIN E

Dr Shute and his colleagues in Canada have shown for over 30 years, the unique role played by this vitamin on circulation and tissue repair. Vitamin E is of specific value in encouraging the uptake of glucose (as glycogen) in the muscles, thus improving the hypoglycaemic symptoms.[57]

VITAMIN C

The vitamin C requirement is often high when the adrenal glands are overworked or exhausted.[58] This vitamin is also of value in normalizing insulin production.

Acupuncture

This ancient therapy is frequently useful in reducing the unpleasant symptoms of low blood sugar. Auricula acupuncture (treating the ear points) is particularly beneficial. In addition to the use of acupuncture needling, some practitioners inject vitamins into the ear points to improve the adrenal efficiency and rebalance the overactive pancreas. (This therapy is referred to as aquapuncture.)[54]

Supplement Recommendations

Although the vitamins and minerals prescribed for hypoglycaemia vary according to the patient's past and present health history, the usual recommendations are as follows. These to be taken daily:

- Vitamin C – 2gm in divided doses.
- Vitamin B-complex (yeast-free) – 50mg of each vitamin.
- Chromium – 500mcgm.
- Magnesium – 500mg.

- Calcium – 500mg.
- Potassium – 250mg.
- Manganese – 10–20mg.
- Pantothenic Acid (vitamin B_5) – 250–500mg.
- Zinc – 25–50mg.
- Vitamin E – 400–500mg.

Note:

1. Vitamin C should be taken in divided doses throughout the day.

2. Vitamin E is only prescribed in high doses if the blood pressure is normal.

3. With selected patients higher doses of various substances are prescribed when indicated. This applies particularly to vitamin E, vitamin B_6, vitamin B_{12}, folic acid and potassium.

Glandular Support

The role of the glandular system has been discussed elsewhere in this book (see Index under Adrenals, Pituitary, Thyroid and Ovaries). Suffice to say that there is frequently a need to prescribe hormone-free tissue concentrates to support failing glands and normalize hormone balance.

Conclusion

As you will begin to understand, the diagnosis and treatment of hypoglycaemia is not a simple matter. The symptoms may be a reflection of serious organic disease, (remember that reactive hypoglycaemia has been called the 'great imitator'). This book is not intended as a treat-yourself manual, and readers are advised to consult a medical *or* non-medical

practitioner who is familiar with the six-hour glucose tolerance test, and understands the symptoms and treatment of
hypoglycaemia. In addition to accurate diagnosis, the treatment needs monitoring, as no two hypoglycaemic patients
are exactly alike. Individual reaction to the diet and other
treatment can vary considerably. Many patients miss the
energy provided by the previous high sugar diet and reassurance and guidance is often needed.

A word here about the need for 'repeat' testing. Very
rarely do I request a second glucose tolerance test. The
taking of neat glucose can cause considerable symptom
aggravation to the hypoglycaemic patient (particularly after
several weeks on the correction diet). The gradual loss of
tenderness over the pancreas, coupled with the improvement
in symptoms, is usually considered sufficient confirmation
that the low blood sugar is normalizing. Repeated testing
may be justified as a research tool, but the clinical priority
is to the patient. It is difficult to justify to the patient the
potential flare-up of symptoms caused by a second GTT,
unless evidence is provided to show it is necessary.

Follow-up Treatment

As I have explained, the diet as outlined earlier in the
chapter is essentially a short-term treatment. Except in very
severe or complicated cases, the diet is prescribed for eight
to twelve weeks. After this time the progress is such that a
follow-up programme is recommended. This involves a diet
consisting of wholewheat bread and cereal, fruit, salads,
vegetables and good quality proteins and fats. Emphasis is
placed on fresh, unrefined foods, and the avoidance of
excesses of any kind. There are, however, still a few 'don'ts'
to follow:

1. Avoid sugar and sugar-rich foods.

2. Avoid caffeine-rich drinks and drugs.

3. Restrict alcohol consumption.

4. Avoid smoking.

5. *Always* have a protein breakfast.

6. Never have a starch-only meal (e.g. bread and cake, cereal and toast).

7. Do not miss meals, particularly important when fatigued or under stress.

There is no need for this type of diet to lead to food fanaticism. The occasional homemade wholemeal cake or biscuits, in the context of a protein meal, should not cause trouble, nor should a glass of dry wine with meals.

If a patient's symptoms gradually return, I advise them to go back on their original diet. With time, most patients learn to understand their own tolerance to starch and sugar and by trial and error find a diet that they are happy with.

The hypoglycaemic diet with its emphasis on low sugar, coffee, tobacco and alcohol is, in many ways, a healthy approach to eating. Often patients find that their whole family (whether hypoglycaemic or not) benefit by following the diet.

Many patients starting the diet are concerned at the possibility of putting on weight (the diet amounts to 2500-3000 calories daily); this fortunately does not seem to happen, indeed most patients actually lose weight. This is not surprising when one realizes that the diet consists of very little carbohydrate, and very little sodium (salt). There is, therefore, a tendency to become more streamlined (owing to fluid loss) without losing a great deal of weight. Fredericks[42] has called this phenomenon 'biochemical spot reducing'.

Problems

For many patients hypoglycaemia is their only problem and a sensible diet with perhaps vitamin and mineral supplements can often produce 100 per cent improvement in health. There are, however, some who do not respond to the diet, although their GTT may confirm low blood sugar, and there are a few patients who actually experience a worsening of symptoms when they change their diet.

The reasons for either lack of response or a temporary adverse response to treatment can be summarized as follows:

1. Although the initial diagnosis may be hypoglycaemia as confirmed with the six-hour test, there may be other factors affecting metabolism and health. It follows that any progress that results from adhering to a low blood sugar correction diet will be in direct proportion to the degree to which the low blood sugar causes the symptoms. For instance, if perhaps 50 per cent of the symptoms can be attributable to low blood sugar, the treatment may only produce a 50 per cent improvement.

2. If the condition is chronic and the patient has suffered for many years other systems of the body may be disturbed, thus reducing the beneficial effects of a dietary change, e.g. adrenal exhaustion owing to chronic stress; liver imbalance owing to obesity or a history of hepatitis, plus

many other health problems including anaemia and hormone imbalance, etc.

3. There may be concurrent food allergies that have been masked by other symptoms, but are greatly aggravated by the high protein-low carbohydrate diet recommended to the low blood sugar sufferer.

4. To influence metabolism by dietary change there are two essential requirements. The diet must be appropriate to the problem and the nutrients must be efficiently digested and absorbed. Many patients have slow or faulty digestive systems and cannot handle the high fat-protein requirements of the hypoglycaemic diet. This problem can, to some extent, be resolved by assessing the patient's metabolic type in terms of slow or fast oxidisers,[59] and their acid or alkaline tendency and prescribing specific vitamin, mineral or digestive enzymes to normalize any imbalance.

5. Many patients feel very tired when they change from a high sugar-caffeine-carbohydrate diet to the hypoglycaemic diet. One simple reason for this is that they miss the instant energy effect of these substances, and their metabolism needs time to adjust to converting the more complex proteins and fats into energy. Until this transition is satisfactorily achieved I recommend that for the first 7-10 days of the diet patients either eat more sweet fruit or take several teaspoonsful of fruit sugar (fructose) throughout the day. The addition of soluble potassium (see page 150) each morning is beneficial as this facilitates the absorption of glucose at cellular level. Protein tablets or drinks between meals can also be beneficial.

6. The ladies as usual have their own special problems when it comes to diagnosing and treating hypoglycaemia. The

chief problems involve the hormone system, in particular the thyroid gland and ovaries. Malfunction of either can cause symptoms that are often confused with the symptoms of hypoglycaemia.

Hypothyroidism

This grand-sounding word means an underactive or sluggish thyroid. The medical word for this deficiency of thyroxin (the thyroid hormone) is myxoedema and is characterized by symptoms of overweight, thickened skin, mental and physical sluggishness and fluid retention. There is also a slow pulse, usually low blood pressure and a coldness of the hands and feet. You may have noted that many of these are also symptoms of hypoglycaemia. To confuse you further, many patients have a slightly underactive thyroid but do *not* have myxoedema. The thyroid is the metabolic pacemaker and, like the choke of a car, it sets the tempo or rate of metabolic activity and influences the speed of metabolism. Quite simply an underactive thyroid slows the body down, and an overactive thyroid speeds the body up. As with many disorders and imbalances in the body there are degrees of malfunction. Pregnancy, stress, incorrect diet, severe infections and surgery can all adversely affect the metabolism and all these factors can influence the delicate thyroid balance. Many women find after childbirth that they have put on weight yet are following their usual diet. They may also be more fatigued with cold hands and feet. Their doctor may suspect a slow thyroid yet their blood tests may not confirm this. The normal-range limits set for thyroid measurements are generally agreed as limits for diagnosing gross under- or over-activity of the gland, and a slight imbalance would not register as abnormal. This explains why many women have symptoms of thyroid deficiency but do not have myxoedema.

As I have said, the metabolism slows down with a slow thyroid and a valuable test that I ask patients to carry out is to measure their body temperature. This is called the Barnes basal temperature test and is widely recommended in America as a more sensitive assessment of hypothyroidism than the standard hospital blood test.[68] The procedure is to check the underarm temperature for ten minutes on waking, for three consecutive mornings. For the women still having periods, the check should be on days 1, 2 and 3 of the period. If the average figure is below 97.8°F there is a good possibility of an underactive thyroid. I have known many patients to have a temperature as low as 95.5°F. The treatment of this problem is aimed at stimulating thyroid activity with a combination of vitamins, minerals, homoeopathic remedies or the use of raw thyroid concentrate (thyroxine-free of bovine source). The gradual rise in the basal temperature coupled with symptom-improvement usually occurs within 3-4 weeks.

Menopause and Oestrogen

No discussion of women's problems and low blood sugar would be complete without mentioning the role played by the menopause, and in particular the hormone oestrogen. Many women between the ages of 35 and 50 have symptoms of low blood sugar, e.g. pre-menstrual tension, fatigue, overweight, depression, migraine, etc., yet when tested low blood sugar is not confirmed with the six-hour GTT and, not surprisingly, they do not respond well to a high protein diet.

Unless a woman has had a total hysterectomy (with removal of the ovaries) the earliest sign of the onset of the menopause and the gradual reduction in oestrogen level, is irregular menstruation either in terms of frequency, duration or heaviness. Some fortunate women find that Hormone Replacement Therapy (HRT) works well, or their own adrenal glands may stimulate the production of oestrogen to support the failing menopausal ovaries. The majority of women, however, with symptoms of fatigue, irritability, headaches, dizziness and depression, and in the age range of 35-50 years, are probably experiencing symptoms of oestrogen deficiency. Other perhaps less obvious symptoms include vaginal infections and dryness, dry skin, breathlessness, chronic cystitis, frequent infections, facial hair, reduction of sex drive and a deepening of the voice. Depression is a very common symptom of the menopausal female and has close links with the oestrogen level. It has been shown that the amino acid Tryptophan (a deficiency of which leads to depression) is deficient in the blood of menopausal females, yet an administration of oestrogen causes a subsequent rise in the tryptophan level.[61] All the symptoms of oestrogen deficiency occur more dramatically and severely following surgical menopause (hysterectomy). A very interesting study carried out by Dr H. Richards in 1973[60] demonstrated that depression following hysterectomy was four times more frequent than normal menopausal depression; in addition, the symptoms were more severe and lasted longer.

Total hysterectomy has been defined as 'a sudden exaggerated menopause' — not without reason. It would seem, however, that when the uterus alone is removed and the ovaries remain, the oestrogen level still drops, possibly owing to impaired circulation or a sympathetic failing of the ovaries following adjacent surgery. When this type of operation is performed the symptoms of oestrogen deficiency may slowly develop 9-12 months after the operation. The medical view that normal oestrogen production continues years after partial or sub-total hysterectomy must be suspect in the light of available evidence.[61] For the female patient with low blood sugar and the practitioner who is treating her, the role of oestrogen and the symptoms of menopause, or post-hysterectomy need to be closely considered, for it is clear that where there is a deficiency, a prescription of a dietary change and vitamin supplements will do little to relieve symptoms, and the patient may simply become more depressed and baffled.

The main orthodox treatment for this problem is HRT. This involves the use of synthetic oestrogen, e.g. the birth pill with all its inherent side-effects, or man-made versions of naturally occurring oestrogen, e.g. *Harmogen*. The natural oestrogen most commonly prescribed – *Premarin* – is extracted and refined from the urine of pregnant mares. In addition to oestrogen, the other female sex hormone, pro-gesterone, is also prescribed. This is mainly used to relieve symptoms of pre-menstrual tension and is prescribed in the UK as *Prempack* or *Duphaston*.

Unfortunately, HRT is not without its side effects which include nausea, headaches, mastitis, weight gain, pigment changes on the face, unexpected bleeding, etc. Fortunately, there are substances widely used in America and recently available in the UK that have many of the benefits of oestrogen and none of the side-effects. These are raw tissue concentrates from animal ovaries, being hormone-free and presented in tablet form. Many other factors are also involved in normal oestrogen production including adrenal and pituitary balance and the optimum availability of many nutrients. For this reason the raw ovary tissue concentrates are usually combined with appropriate vitamins, minerals and raw tissue extracts of pituitary, adrenals and thyroid.

Summary

If patients with symptoms of low blood sugar and a diagnosis confirmed by a six-hour GTT do not show a reasonably good response to the dietary change and vitamin and mineral supplementation within 4-6 weeks I follow the simple rule — LOOK AGAIN. There may be a thyroid imbalance, an oestrogen deficiency, severe stress leading to adrenal exhaustion, liver imbalance, poor digestion with faulty absorption, a masked food allergy or candiasis. I always make a point of explaining to patients that although they would appear to have low blood sugar it may not be their *only* problem, and if their progress is not satisfactory, further tests may be necessary. These tests could involve additional blood tests, hair analysis or a detailed investigation of suspect food or environmental allergies. Low blood sugar may be the chief cause of such symptoms, but it may also be a symptom of a more deep-rooted and as yet undiagnosed cause.

GLOSSARY

Acetone Substance found in urine in fasting. Released in excessive quantities in the urine and breath of uncontrolled diabetics.

Acidosis Said to occur when the compensatory mechanisms of overbreathing and creation of very acid urine are 'stretched to the limit' and drowsiness or coma occur. Ketone substances are present in the blood.

Adrenal Glands Paired glands, also called the suprarenal glands, located adjacent to the tip of each kidney.

Adrenal Cortex Outer layer of the adrenal gland – secretes the steroid hormones including cortisone.

Adrenal Medulla Central part of the adrenal gland – secretes adrenaline.

Adrenalin Hormone produced by the adrenal glands to facilitate sudden physical activity in emergency. One effect of adrenalin is to increase blood sugar.

Aetiology The causation of disease.

Allergen Substance which causes tissue to become sensitive.

Atherosclerosis Narrowing of blood vessels.

Aura Sensation, auditory or visual, experiences by patient prior to epileptic or migraine attack.

Calorie The amount of heat required to raise temperature of one gram of water by 1°C. The total amount of heat available from full combustion of food is: from carbohydrate 4.1 Kcal/g, from protein 4.3 Kcal/g, from fat 9.0 Kcal/g. N.B. in nutritional and metabolic studies the Kilo calorie is generally abbreviated to Calorie but written with a capital C to indicate that it is the larger unit.

Carbohydrate Energy-producing compounds of carbon, oxygen and hydrogen; (starch, sugar, glucose etc.).

Citric Acid Cycle See **Krebs Cycle**.

Cortisol Substance similar to cortisone released by the adrenal glands; also called hydro-cortisone.

Cortisone A carbohydrate/protein-regulating hormone, released by the adrenal glands.

Cranial Nerves A group of 12 pairs of nerves connected with the brain. These include the optic, trigeminal and vagus nerves.

Dumping Syndrome A condition due to gastric surgery, where the stomach contents rapidly empty, producing a sudden elevation of blood sugar.

Dysinsulinism Term implying disturbance of normal insulin-production. May therefore result in a combination of high and low blood sugar, usually considered to be pre-diabetic.

EEG Electroencephalogram – a record of the electrical currents developed by the brain.

Endocrine Means literally secreted internally, applied to substances produced and released into the blood, especially hormones.

Endogenous Arising from or growing from within; or arising from causes within an organism.

Enzyme Substances produced by the body, acting as a catalyst by increasing reactions of various substances.

Epinephrine Term used in the USA for Adrenalin.

Fructose Fruit sugar also called levulose, found in all sweet fruits.

Functional Hypoglycaemia Hyperinsulinism — see **Reactive Hypoglycaemia**.

Glandular Extracts Nutritional supplements derived from animal glands or organs. They are usually in tablet form and combined with synergistic vitamin and mineral support. Specific glandular disfunction or weakness can be supported with these extracts, such as thyroid, adrenal, ovary.

Glycogen A polysaccharide, the main carbohydrate storage material in man, formed by and largely stored in the liver; also stored in muscle. Known also as 'animal starch'.

Growth Hormone Substance that stimulates growth mainly secreted by pituitary gland, exerts direct effect on protein, carbohydrate and fat metabolism.

GTT Glucose Tolerance Test.

Hair Mineral Analysis This diagnostic method is used to analyse trace minerals in human hair. Approximately one gram of hair is sufficient to yield figures on 27-30 trace amounts of both essential and toxic minerals. These figures closely reflect mineral reserves in muscle and liver tissue.

Haemophilia Congenital tendency to haemorrhage, owing to impaired clotting ability. Occurs only in males.

Hidden Sugar Sugar in foods, see Table 3 for examples.

Histamine Substance found in the body, released after injury, also concerned with the control of tissue permeability.

Histaminase Substance produced by the liver, acts by inactivating histamine.

Hydro-Cortisone See **Cortisol**.

Hyperinsulinism See **Reactive Hypoglycaemia**.

'Hypo' Effect Hypoglycaemia produced in the diabetic patient owing to excess insulin dosage.

Hypothesis A supposition, assumed as a basis of reasoning.

Idiopathic Self-originating, of unknown cause. Used to describe disease of spontaneous origin.

Insulin Hormone released by the Islet glands of the pancreas to control the level of sugar in the blood.

Islets of Langerhans Small glands in the pancreas producing insulin.

Ketogenic Diet High fat/protein diet; prescribed to encourage weight loss through breakdown of body's fat reserves.

Ketones Acetones and allied substances resulting from breakdown of fats.

Ketosis See **Acidosis**.

Krebs Cycle The final process or pathway whereby food is broken down, being converted to energy; carbon dioxide and water.

Lactose Milk sugar: breaks down to galactose and glucose.

Molasses Thick sweet syrup, residue remaining after crystalization of sugar. Contains sucrose, fructose, calcium, potassium and many B vitamins.

Monosaccharides Simplest sugar, e.g. glucose.

Neuroglycopenia Symptoms produced as a result of reduction of glucose supply to nerve tissue.

Oedema Abnormal amount of fluid in tissue; causing swelling and puffiness.

Pancreas Gland situated left upper abdomen, secretes digestive enzymes and insulin (also known as sweetbreads).

Pellagra Deficiency of vitamin B_3 (nicotinic acid) causing dementia, diarrhoea and dermatitis.

Pituitary Gland Master gland situated in skull; produces substances that influence thyroid, adrenals, growth, gonads and fluid balance.

Phospholipid Fat-containing phosphorus, e.g. lecithin.

Physiology The study of processes that occur in living system.

Polysaccharide Carbohydrates containing more than two basic single sugar units in their molecule, e.g. starch, glycogen.

Psychosomatic Relating to both mind and body.

Reactive Hypoglycaemia Hypoglycaemia due to body's over-reaction to sugar. Also called 'hyperinsulinism'.

Relative Hypoglycaemia See **Reactive Hypoglycaemia**.

Renal Diabetes Diabetes thought to be dependent on defective kidney function.

Renal Threshold Concentration of a substance in the blood at which it appears in the urine.

Rickets Deficiency of calcium availability to bones, usually due to vitamin D deficiency.

Saccharine Disease Term used by T. L. Cleeve to define conditions caused by the taking of refined starch and sugar, e.g. coronary disease, peptic ulcer, etc.

Scurvy Vitamin C deficiency, symptoms include haemorrhage of gums and swelling of tissue.

Starch Carbohydrates made up of a chain of monosaccharide sugars, i.e. polysaccharides.

Sucrose Disaccharide (double sugar); the molecule contains two basic simple sugar units known as cane or beet sugar.

Thyroid Gland Gland located anterior throat. Secretes thyroxine which controls metabolism, growth and development.

Thyrotoxicosis Hyperthyroidism, condition caused by

excess production of thyroxine; leading to weight loss, rapid heart, etc.

Thyroxine See **Thyroid Gland**.

Trace Elements Mineral substances, present in the body in minute amounts, necessary for good health, e.g. cobalt, manganese, etc.

Transient Hypoglycaemia Temporary low blood sugar, usually due to exercise, fatigue or missed meals. Usually reversible without treatment.

Trigeminal Neuralgia Facial pain confined to branches of the trigeminal nerve (one of the cranial nerves).

Triglycerides Stored body fat; derived from the diet or synthesized in the liver.

Vagal Pertaining to the vagus nerve.

Vagus Nerve One of the 12 cranial nerves, influences digestion. This is effected during migraine attacks.

Vasodilation Dilation of blood vessels.

Where to seek help

The six-hour GTT is not a standard hospital test. For this and other reasons, most GPs are not familiar with the diagnosis and treatment of reactive hypoglycaemia. Those who are, are usually in the private sector of health care. Practitioners of complementary medicine; naturopaths, herbalists, acupuncturists, homoeopaths and osteopaths, are more aware of hypoglycaemia and are therefore more likely to know which of their colleagues use the GTT on a regular basis. Very few practitioners in Great Britain test their patients for hypoglycaemia with the six-hour GTT. For further information and practitioners' names write to the following, enclosing a stamped self-addressed envelope:

The Bournemouth Complementary Medical Practice
Ridge Cottage
29 Ferncroft Road
Dorset
BH10 6BY

REFERENCES

1 Zieva and Pannall. *Clinical Chemistry in Diagnosis and Treatment*, pp. 270-5 (Lloyd-Luke Ltd., 1975).
2 E. A. Graham and N. A. Womack, 'Surgery of Hypoglycaemia', *Pract. Med. Ser.*, 1933.
— 'Application of Surgery to Hypoglycaemic State due to Islet Tumors of Pancreas and other Conditions', *Surg. Gynae and Obstec.*, 1933, pp. 728–42.
3 Seale Harris, 'The Diagnosis and Treatment of Hyperinsulinism', *Ann. Intern. Med.*, 10, 1936.
4 M. Fabrykant, *Metabolism*, Vol. 4, 1955.
5 D. Anthony, 'Personality Disorders and Reactive Hypoglycaemia', *Diabetes*, Vol. 22, 9, pp. 664–75, 1973.
6 D. Anthony, 'Hypoglycaemia and Personality', *B.M.J.*, 20 April, 1974.
7 W. E. Beebe and O.W. Wendell, 'Preliminary Observations of Altered Carbohydrate Metabolism in Psychiatric Patients' in *Orthomolecular Psychiatry*, edited by Hawkins and Pauling (W. H. Freeman, 1973).
8 P. L. Meiers, 'Relative Hypoglycaemia in Schizophrenia' in *Orthomolecular Psychiatry*, edited by Hawkins and Pauling (W. H. Freeman, 1973).

9 Seale Harris, 'Hyperinsulinism and Dysinsulinism', *Journal American Medical Association*, Vol. 83, 1924.

10 John Yudkin, *Pure White and Deadly* (Davis-Poynter, 1972).

11 H. J. Roberts, *New England Journal of Medicine*, 268, 562, 1963.

12 James Wilkinson, *Daily Express*, 31 July 1968.

13 E. P. Joslin, *Diabetes Mellitus* (Lea and Febiger, 1971).

14 H. Kaplan, *Annals of Allergy*, 21, 41, 1963.

15 Malcolm I. V. Jayson and Allan Dixon, *Rheumatism and Arthritis* (Pan Books, 1974).

16 Hans Seyle, *The Stress of Life* (McGraw, 1978).

17 Roger Williams, *Nutrition Against Disease* (Bantam, 1973).

18 E. M. Abrahamson and A. W. Pezet, *Body Mind and Sugar* (Holt, Rinehart and Winston, 1951).

19 W. Philpott, *New Dynamics of Preventive Medicine*, Vol. 1, 1974.

20 Mandell and Scanlon, *Dr Mandell's 5-Day Allergy Relief System* (Arrow Books, 1983).

21 Randolf and Moss, *Allergies* (Turnstone Press, 1980).

22 Arthur Coca, *The Pulse Test* (Lyle Stuart, New York, 1967).

23 Bryan and Bryan, 'The Application of In Vitro Cytotoxic Reactions in the Clinical Diagnosis of Food Allergy', *Laryngoscope* LXX, 6, pp. 810-24, 1960.

24 'Cytotoxic Reactions in the Diagnosis of Food Allergy' A.L.R.O.S., 72nd A.G.M., March 1969. (Holt, Rinehart and Winston, 1951).

25 *National Health Interview Survey*, 1966/67, US Dept. of Health, Education and Welfare.

26 E. Cheraskin and W. M. Ringsdorf, *Psychodietetics* (Bantam, 1976).

27 Dr R. C. Atkins and S. M. Linde, *Dr Atkins Super Energy Diet* (Corgi, 1979).

28 T. L. Cleave, *The Saccharine Disease* (Wright, Bristol, 1974).

29 Dr R. Ahrens, *The American Journal of Clinical Nutrition*, Vol. 27, 1974.

30 Dr B. Sandler, *Homoeostasis*, Autumn 1974.

31 Roger Williams, *Biochemical Individuality* (University of Texas Press, 1970).

32 L. D. Lewis et al, 'Cerebral Energy State in Insulin-Induced Hypoglycaemia Related to Blood Glucose and to E.E.G.', *Journal of Neuro-Chemistry*, Vol. 23, 1974.

33 L. D. Lewis et al, 'Changes in Carbohydrate Substances, Amino Acids and Ammonia in the Brain during Insulin-Induced Hypoglycaemia', *Journal of Neuro-Chemistry*, Vol. 23, 1974.

34 B. T. Burton, *Heinz Handbook of Nutrition*, (McGraw, 1976).

35 E. Cheraskin, 'Cancer Proneness Profile', *Geriatrics*, August 1969.

36 J. F. Greder, 'Anxiety and Caffeinism: A Diagnostic Dilemma', *American Journal of Psychiatry*, 131 (10), pp. 1089-92, Oct. 1974.

37 L. K. Altman, *New York Times*, 15 March, 1975.

38 D. Cairns, C. W. Deveney et al, 'Mechanism of Release of Gastrin by Insulin Hypoglycaemia', *Surgical Forum*, Vol. 25, 1974.

39 G. Feurle, R. Arnold et al, 'Rise in Serum Gastrin during Insulin Hypoglycaemia with and without Simultaneous Gastric Aspiration', *German Medicine*, Vol. 3, 1973.

40 T. L. Cleave, *The Peptic Ulcer* (Bristol, Wright, 1962).

41 *Prevention*, Vol. 23, No.5, May 1980.

42 C. Fredericks and H. Goodman, *Low Blood Sugar and You*, (Constellation International, 1969).

43 Paavo Airola, *Hypoglycaemia – A Better Approach* (Health Plus Publishers, 1974).

44 J. Quartermain, Report Roulett Inst. 24. 100, 1968.

45 H. H. Sandstead et al, *Zinc Metabolism* (Ed. A. S. Prasad), p. 304 (C. C. Thomas, Springfield).

46 I. J. T. Davies, *The Clinical Significance of the Essential Biological Metals* (Heinemann Med., 1972).

47 H. A. Schroder, *Journal of Nutrition*, Vol. 94, 1968b.

48 L. A. Maynard et al, *Journal of Nutrition*, Vol. 64, 1958.

49 D. H. P. Streeten et al, *Journal of Physiology*, Vol. 118, 1952.

50 E. S. Egeli et al, *American Heart Journal*, Vol. 95, 1960.

51 H. F. West, *The Lancet*, 2, 877, 1958.

52 B. H. Ershoff et al, *Journal of Nutrition* Vol. 50, 1953.

53 R. E. Hodges et al, *Journal of Clinical Investigations* Vol. 38, 1959.

54 W. H. Khoe, 'The Treatment of Functional Hypoglycaemia with Acupuncture and Diet', *American Journal of Acupuncture*, Vol. 3, No. 4, Oct/Dec 1975.

55 H. R. V. Arnstein and R. J. Wrighton (Eds), *The Cobalamins* A Glaxo Symposium (Churchill Livingstone, 1970).

56 Adelle Davies, *Let's Get Well* (Allen and Unwin, 1966).

57 W. E. Shute, Complete Updated Vitamin E Book (Keats, 1975).

58 B. H. Ershoff, *Nut. Rev.*, Vol. 13, No. 33, 1955.

59 George Watson, *Nutrition and Your Mind* (Souvenir Press, 1974).

60 Dr D. H. Richards, 'Depression and Menopause', *The Lancet*, August 1973.

61 Wendy Cooper, *No Change* (Arrow Books, 1983).

62 Gay Gaer Luce, *Body Time* (Paladin, 1974), pp. 120-1.

63 Arabella Boxer, *Mediterranean Cookbook* (Penguin, 1983).

64 Gilly Smith & Rowena Goldman, *The Mediterranean Health Diet* (Headline, 1993).

65 Carol & Malcolm McConnell, *The Mediterranean Diet* (Bodley Head, 1987).

66 Claudia Roden, *Mediterranean Cookbook* (BBC Books, 1989).

67 Martin & Maggie Budd, *Recipes for Health: Low Blood Sugar* (Thorsons, 1995).

68 Broda D. Barnes, *Hypothyroidism: The Unsuspected Illness* (Harper & Row, 1976).

69 Martin Budd, 'Hypoglycaemia and Personality' *Complementary Therapies in Medicine* (1994), 2, pp. 144–6.

INDEX